change your habits, change your life

change your habits, change your life

A Proven Plan for Healthy Living

DANNA DEMETRE

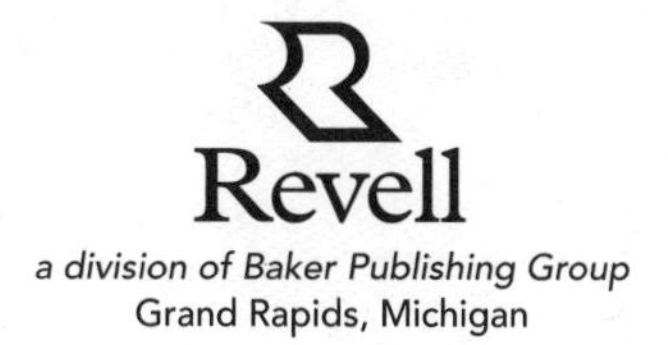

a division of Baker Publishing Group
Grand Rapids, Michigan

Published by Revell
a division of Baker Publishing Group
P.O. Box 6287, Grand Rapids, MI 49516-6287
www.revellbooks.com

Printed in the United States of America

Library of Congress Cataloging-in-Publication Data

Demetre, Danna.
Change your habits, change your life : a proven plan for healthy living / Danna Demetre.
p. cm.
Includes bibliographical references.
ISBN 978-0-8007-3331-5 (pbk.)
1. Health—Religious aspects—Christianity. 2. Food habits. 3. Habit breaking—Religious aspects—Christianity. 4. Change (Psychology)—Religious aspects—Christianity. I. Title.
BT732.D45 2009
248.8′6—dc22 2008041927

Portions of this book are from Danna Demetre's book *Scale Down: A Realistic Guide to Balancing Body, Soul, and Spirit* (Grand Rapids: Revell, 2003).

This is a book based on the research of the author, and the ideas, procedures, and suggestions in this book are not intended as a substitute for the medical advice of your personal health professional. All matters regarding your health require medical supervision. Consult your physician before adopting any of the suggestions in this book (whether or not explicitly noted in the text), as well as about any condition that may require diagnosis or medical attention. In addition, the statements made by the author regarding certain products or services represent the opinion of the author alone and do not constitute a recommendation or endorsement of any product or service by the publisher. The author and publisher disclaim any liability arising directly or indirectly from the use of the book or any products mentioned herein.

Published in association with the literary agency of Alive Communications, Inc. 7680 Goddard Street, Suite 200, Colorado Springs, CO 80920. www.alivecommunications.com.

In keeping with biblical principles of creation stewardship, Baker Publishing Group advocates the responsible use of our natural resources. As a member of the Green Press Initiative, our company uses recycled paper when possible. The text paper of this book is comprised of 30% post-consumer waste.

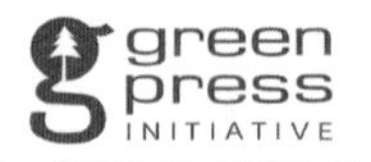

contents

introduction

What's Wrong with Me?

"What's wrong with me? I can't even make it one day without giving into my cravings and going on a binge. I feel like food has total control over me. Will I struggle like this the rest of my life? Why can't I just be normal and eat when I'm hungry? I'm a total loser. I'll never change."

Most evenings this young nursing student found herself hanging over the toilet bowl vomiting after she'd binged on doughnuts, cookies, potato chips, or whatever else she could accumulate quickly on her embarrassing daily raid of the local mini-mart on the way home from classes. Tonight she ended her purging session sobbing into the porcelain bowl. "Why can't I stop this?" No one answered her pathetic plea.

She'd been struggling for almost five years, and no one knew. While she could stand to lose fifteen or twenty pounds, she looked fairly good in her clothes. Most people called her pretty. She seemed smart, secure, and well liked. She *was* well liked by everyone but herself.

Now she was engaged to a man nine years her senior who said he would not marry her until she weighed 120 pounds. She thought that his demand would be great motivation, but it only sent her into a more dangerous cycle. Now, she was considering taking amphetamines again to kill her insatiable appetite. She knew better. But, how could pills be worse than what she was doing to her body—sometimes bingeing and purging up to five times a day? She believed her own lie and found an old friend from high school who still had "connections."

The pills worked great. She had no appetite and great energy. The "speed" made her restless when she sat studying for hours, so she took up smoking to give herself something to do. As soon as she lost all the weight, she'd give up the cigarettes and the pills. She knew she'd have the motivation once she was thin. (That's what they all say.)

She was more on task with her studies and feeling great as the pounds dropped off faster than ever. She'd be married in no time! And she was. She took her scale on her honeymoon. She just had to maintain that 120 pounds, fearing the rejection of her new husband if she didn't. A few days into her marriage, she flushed the diet pills down the toilet, vowing to never take them again. She had to stop. She had no choice. She was beginning to have really scary panic attacks. Her appetite returned. The panic attacks got worse.

After several months of unrelenting fear, she called on her husband more and more to assure her she would be okay. But he was confused and repulsed by her anxiety and simply withdrew. So once again . . . she ate . . . and ate . . . and ate. And she purged. He never knew her secret. He only knew that she didn't have the perfect 120-pound body anymore. She had the average 148-pound one that he loathed . . . that she loathed too. She felt lost, trapped, weak, and afraid. Afraid she could never change and be the healthy woman inside and out she so desired to be.

That young woman was me—over thirty years ago. I had some dangerously unhealthy habits that were firmly supported by some dangerously unhealthy thinking. What started as occasional overeating led to compulsive overeating, and then in my desire to control my out-of-control behavior, I resorted to purging. That dangerous habit of bulimia peaked in college but actually continued intermittently for about sixteen years.

I share all of this with you because I want you to know that I know what it feels like to be in bondage. I thought the problem was all about my behavior. I discovered that in reality it was all about my unhealthy beliefs and thought patterns. My journey out of bondage took a while because I tried for many years to change from the outside in. I changed my behavior, hoping it would change my urges. That really never worked for long. I'd lose a few pounds, or quit smoking for a few weeks, only to return to my old habits, feeling more defeated and pathetic than ever.

The victory I finally found was not really of my own doing. And it certainly wasn't in the order I would have chosen. You see, those panic attacks became so unrelenting that I literally thought I was losing my mind . . . dying . . . or both. The unremitting anxiety led me to seek help, first from medical doctors, then from counselors and psychiatrists. I was the ultimate hypochondriac for a few years, sure that the medical doctors were missing some hidden disease that was going to kill me at any moment. I was so motivated to discover my malady that I got straight As in my medical-surgical classes and then again in my psychology unit. But all that study left me still wondering, *What's wrong with me? And, if I do die, what will become of me?*

One night, I felt like I was being consumed by a dark fog, my fear so paralyzing that I could barely breathe. A thought came to mind: *No one can help me. I'm all alone in this dark tunnel, lost with no way out and no human being can show me the way. Only God, if he cares, can help me out of this darkness.* The problem was, I didn't know where to find God. I grew up in a great home with loving, supportive parents but without any religious faith. I had been to church only a few times in my entire life. I believed that God existed, but I had no idea how to find him.

There is a Scripture (Jer. 29:11–14) that says:

> "For I know the plans I have for you," declares the Lord, "plans to prosper you and not to harm you, plans to give you hope and a future.

> Then you will call upon me and come and pray to me, and I will listen to you. You will seek me and find me when you seek me with all your heart. I will be found by you," declares the LORD.

In my naivety I sought God with all my heart. As promised, I found him and realized that he knew everything about me. And most importantly, I learned that he loved me despite my failures, or what those Christians called sin.

A woman I barely knew shared the good news about Jesus with me. Tonette explained that I was separated from God (who is perfect and holy) because of my sin. She said I was not alone, that everyone has sinned (even people like Billy Graham), and that everyone falls short of God's standard. But God in his great love chose to come to the earth in the person of Jesus Christ—all man and all God—for the sole purpose of dying for my sins, well, actually, everyone's sins. But at that moment I was only worried about me! (If you want to know more about a personal relationship with Christ, please turn to page 345 at the end of this book.)

As strange as the message was to me, I somehow knew deep in my soul that it was true. And even though I did not understand everything about God and sin, I knew in my spirit that God was drawing me near and that he did have all the answers to my wretched life. And the extra bonus was that this forgiveness not only gave me access to God right now in this life but secured eternal life with him as well. How cool is that?

Well, being a typical type A kind of gal, I was truly hoping that God would give me an immediate healing of my panic attacks and bulimia, and while he was at it, maybe even cure me of my smoking habit. He did cure me, but not immediately. In the months and years that followed, God took me on an incredible journey of transformation. In Romans 12:2 it says,

> Do not conform any longer to the pattern of this world, but be transformed by the renewing of your mind.

I desired above anything to be totally renewed and transformed. But I had no idea where to begin. So, I simply prayed for God to show me the way, and he did. He taught me many powerful truths about how he designed the human mind and most importantly the power of his Word to replace the lies I believed with truth. It is my heart's desire to pass on what I learned to you.

Over time, I was completely healed of my panic attacks without drugs or therapy. I quit smoking, never to be tempted again. And, I not only overcame my greatest and longest battle of all, my bulimia, but I found complete victory over food and an unhealthy body image. I'll tell you more about how this all unfolded later.

The reason I am writing this book is because far too many people have never found lasting victory over their destructive thinking, which is at the root of all bad habits. (Note: physical addictions to things like nicotine or narcotics must be dealt with in addition to unhealthy thinking.) The truths I will share with you are actually effective in all areas of your life. Whenever you believe a persistent lie, I can assure you that negative emotions and damaging behaviors will follow. To find lasting and complete victory, you must identify the lies and replace them with truth. I'll explain how to do just that in chapter 2.

In my first book, *Scale Down: A Realistic Guide to Balancing Body, Soul, and Spirit*, I wrote about the battle of the mind in addition to the physical principles necessary to acquire a lean, healthy body for life without dieting. Those principles have helped thousands learn how to lose weight by making lifestyle changes they can maintain for a lifetime. I know from uncountable emails that my teaching struck a chord.

Yet, I believe there is a need for more in-depth teaching and guidance in the area of renewing the mind. It is simply too easy to put undue focus on behavior and neglect the underlying cause of your habits—destructive beliefs. I can assure you that I will certainly address the number one bad habit in America—overeating. But I will also address all aspects of healthy living. The quality of our life is contingent on how we feel. And unless you come from a unique gene pool that allows you to live poorly and still feel great, you need to learn how to eat, exercise, rest, and de-stress in ways that promote vitality.

Who Will This Book Help?

Some of you may be thin, but unless you have truly "arrived" with a lifestyle that is consistently healthy, this book is for you. Many of you are not experiencing the level of bondage that I experienced. Some of you are. No matter. If you want to learn how to have victory in all the dimensions of your life—victory that honors God and brings you great peace—this book is for you.

And lest I sound like I have fully arrived myself, let me confess. I have not. But, I am a pretty good role model, living and eating, moving and sleeping, in ways that promote good health most of the time. The older I get, the more dedicated I am to "doing the right things" so I can finish strong and enjoy my children and grandchildren as long as the Lord keeps me here on earth.

Change . . . Change . . . Change

Did you notice that the word *change* shows up two times in the title of this book? If I had it my way, it would actually show up three times—because we need to change our mind, which in turn changes our habits, which ultimately changes our life. But for book covers, a long title is difficult to grasp, so we address all three "changes" within the body of the book, and you'll understand after reading that the changed habits are actually an outflow of changed minds.

Isn't that what you really want to experience . . . lasting, victorious change? As I've already said—and I really want you to "get" this—too often we try to change only our behavior and wonder why it is such a struggle to stay on track. While behavioral change is necessary, without the lasting foundation of a renewed mind, you will fall back into your old habits sooner than later.

So, we will work on both your mind and your behavior together for the next forty days. I will be your virtual coach—teaching, encouraging, and prodding you on day after day. I only wish that I could have had a coach that addressed my body, soul, and spirit when I was struggling. I hope that you find the initial teaching chapters followed by our daily journey (which includes devotional, health facts, journal, and logging sections) a strong support as you move closer and closer to a permanently transformed mind. And when the mind changes, watch out . . . your behavior will always follow!

PART I

a foundation for change

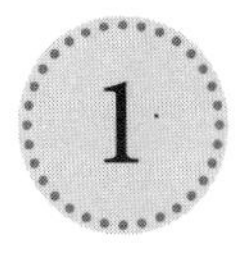

the dynamics of change

High school reunions . . . they bring back so many memories—and bring out so many unexpected emotions. I just went to my husband's thirtieth this past summer, and I was shocked. There were so many really *old* people there! Seriously, many of the men and women seemed old beyond their years . . . and unhealthy. Now, I'm not one of those "younger" wives. I'm actually seven years older than my husband. (Yes, sadly, my first marriage ended in divorce after eleven years.) I'm not trying to be supercritical, but the reason I bring up this observation is because it occurred to me that the years just fly by, and before we know it, we are "wearing" our habits, so to speak.

How you take care of yourself every day makes a huge difference in your health, vitality, and appearance. It's so easy to let our little unhealthy habits carry on and on, year after year, thinking we will make a change . . .

when work isn't so busy . . .
when the holidays are over . . .
when we have a little more money . . .
when we're not so tired . . .

When . . . when . . . when . . . never comes. Well, this book is about making "when" . . . *now*. As I've already said, it will be a simplified guide to changing your old, unhealthy habits one day at a time by changing your mind. And, if you will follow it the best you can (not perfectly—just consistently) for the next forty days, I truly believe you can change your life in important ways. That being said, I must be honest and disclose these realities up front:

change is difficult
change is simple
change takes time

Perhaps at first glance you may find these statements rather confusing and contradictory. Let me explain.

Change is difficult because too often we approach it all wrong. We begin by trying to change our behavior with our eyes focused on the goal of losing weight, getting healthier, gaining fitness, and the like. That sounds like the right approach, doesn't it? But if it is, then why do most people who try to lose weight, stop smoking, or change any habit rarely succeed long term? I believe it is because they attempt to change from the outside in rather than from the inside out. I want to encourage you to try something new this time . . . thinking first and acting second.

When we take the "inside out" approach by changing our thinking, our behavior will eventually (and naturally) follow. That is *if* (and that is a big *if*) we practice that new thinking long enough.

Change is simple when we identify the unhealthy thinking that drives our behavior and give ourselves new, productive, and renewing messages.

Change takes time because God designed our brains with a protective mechanism that requires consistent repetition before any dynamic change can occur. I'll tell you more about how that works later. And of course, the actual physical changes take as long as they take. I'm sorry if that sounds flippant. But quite frankly, wouldn't you like to make this change once and for all and be done with it, even if it takes six months, a year, or longer, rather than go at it again and again and never find true victory?

The Outside Still Counts

The "inside out" approach does not neglect the fact that we must begin to implement healthier behaviors even before our mind is totally transformed by new perspectives. In this journey, I will give you many simple principles that you will "practice" until they become natural. No matter what habit is your greatest enemy, we will address your total body and all its needs in very realistic ways. But to clarify, I am not going to go into lengthy explanations about nutrition, exercise, and so forth. I've written extensively on those topics in *Scale Down*. Rather, I am going to remind you of what you probably already know about eating healthy, daily exercising, diminishing stress, and getting adequate rest. I will do so by giving you some body "word pictures," new perspectives, and compelling motivations to catch your attention until your mind catches up.

Celebrate Each Small Step

The journey toward gaining (and maintaining) a lean, healthy body can be long and sometimes difficult. It took me many years to get to the place where I felt completely out of bondage to food. Yet, as I look back, there were many lasting, positive changes along the way that I failed to celebrate fully. Instead of focusing on the small steps I was consistently making, I would tend to dwell on the occasional step backward. If you are doing better than you were last year, then that is great cause for celebration.

Unfortunately, most of us measure our progress in black-and-white terms. We are either on a diet or off a diet. We are exercising regularly or we are not exercising at all. We are controlling our habit or we are letting our habit control us. We have more than enough information to succeed. In fact, we've become experts on the areas in which we are challenged. Yet, despite all the head knowledge, we struggle to put what we know into practice and achieve lasting success.

Is Anybody Succeeding Out There?

The Internet is a wonderful thing. I just finished searching dozens of websites that shared hundreds of weight loss stories. I love to read about how people have succeeded at losing significant amounts of weight. Every diet and program has its stories. Yet, I always get a little discouraged because I know the sad reality. Most of those "successes" will consider themselves failures in less than a year.

I am passionate about helping others find permanent solutions that honor God. I am really not a weight loss guru, though I have many opinions about losing weight healthfully. If anything, I'm a "biblical change coach." I believe God has provided us powerful insights in his Word as to how we can change in every area of life. I'm not revealing any new secrets. God doesn't keep secrets from us. His Word speaks specifically to the battle of the flesh and the battle of the mind. If we read and apply his principles, we can become fully transformed. That is why the byline of this book is "a *proven* plan for healthy living." God's precepts are perfect and proven ways to live with victory in all dimensions of life . . . if only we follow them.

> "Don't even try to tell me the latest, greatest weight loss secret. I'm an expert at weight loss. I've lost and gained the same twenty pounds dozens of times!" ~ Anonymous

Just *Don't* Do It

Have you ever considered that changing most habits (except perhaps the habit of being a couch potato) requires very little or no action? In fact, the opposite is true. Changing a habit is more about doing nothing at all. For example, when dealing with the habit of overeating or indulging in unhealthy foods, the change needed most is to simply stop eating too much unhealthy food. When it comes to smoking, drinking alcohol, gambling, or even shopping too much, the same is true. You don't need to *do* anything—but rather stop doing those activities that are negatively impacting your life. It sounds so simple; just *don't* do it.

Yet, those of us who have struggled with a bad habit know it's not that easy. It often feels like we are literally programmed to carry out the same unhealthy behaviors over and over like robots. And that's because . . . we are programmed. After months, years, sometimes decades of practicing unhealthy habits, we have developed an autopilot response that is buried deep in the neuron pathways of our brain. So, it's time to learn (or relearn) how to biblically and healthfully reprogram yourself toward healthy thinking and living.

A Personal Coach

As I said earlier in this chapter, change is simple. We don't need a huge amount of information. But, I do think we all need an opportunity to walk alongside someone who has found victory. Following are four chapters that will lay a foundation so our daily "sessions" are more effective. It is important to read those chapters before officially starting your forty-day journey. Then, you just take one day at a time, starting with day 1, until you complete day 40. If you must skip a day (due to death or illness . . . or some other grand excuse), then pick up where you left off as soon as you possibly can. However, except for extreme circumstances, don't take any breaks. Once you've read the first chapters, your daily reading, logging, and brief journaling will only take ten to twenty minutes.

A Journey to the Future

In closing this chapter, I'd like you to take a brief imaginary journey. We are going to fast-forward to exactly one year from today. In this future time, you are sitting here rereading this paragraph and thinking about how far you have come in one short year. You can see yourself as you were one year ago. It's hard to believe that you struggled so long and yet you have come so far. You love the victory you have experienced over your old unhealthy habits. You love the way your body, soul, and spirit have responded to your new healthy attitudes. You feel more energized and alive than you ever have before. You embrace the awesome plans that God has for your life and welcome each new day with joy. You never believed you could finally cross over to such a place, but now you know what it means to be "transformed by the renewing of your mind."

change your mind

My heart was racing so fast I thought it would pound right out of my chest. I was trying to stay focused, but it was hard to catch my breath. My sense of sight and sound was heightened, yet somehow oddly distorted. The lights were too bright, the sounds too loud. It felt like I was on sensory overload with everything around me rising to an intolerable level. All I wanted to do was get my groceries out of the basket and through the checkout before I lost my mind. Was that so hard?

Actually, it was painfully difficult. And I simply could not complete the task. With all of my items still spread out on the counter, I ran out of the store, leaving the poor clerk to deal with my stuff.

I sat in the privacy and security of my car, my face in my hands, trying to slow my breathing, wanting desperately to feel the air drawing into my lungs. But, as with most of my panic attacks, I felt like I was suffocating . . . even dying. I was in a constant battle to remain sane and alive—a battle waged entirely in my own mind.

Five years of fear is torture. My battle with bulimia and body image paled in comparison to the all-encompassing war that I was fighting for survival. And yet, despite my fear of dying or going crazy, I still ran to food between my panic attacks. That is, until one day when I finally began seeking God. And as I've already shared, I found him. That very first day, he began to transform me. It began with a daily renewing of my mind.

As a new believer, I had no concept of spiritual truth beyond the fact that I was a sinner and Jesus Christ died for my sins. But, I later learned that when we open our heart to God and trust in Christ alone for our salvation, he sends his Holy Spirit to take residence in us. I didn't even understand this profound truth intellectually, but I completely sensed it in my spirit. I just knew that I would never be alone again. That one simple fact gave me hope and courage.

Never Alone

When my panic attacks continued, I did not think that God had left me or was waiting for me to jump through all sorts of hoops to prove myself to him. I just sensed that he was teaching me to trust him. And he was. So, when a panic attack would begin to overcome me, I started to respond differently. First, I would not let myself "run" like I did at the grocery store and so many other places. Second, and most important, I started telling myself a new message. I would say things to myself such as, *God is with me; I'm never alone. He will help me get through this. Hey, I never died before, and I'm not going to die now. And when I do die, at least I know where I am going!*

Within a few days of reading the Bible, I ran across the most incredible verse, and it seemed like God was speaking directly to my heart. "For God has not given us a spirit of fear, but of power and of love and of a sound mind" (2 Tim. 1:7 NKJV). Those words completely resonated in my soul. I felt like I had just discovered a treasure of great worth. And I had.

The Power of Truth

Every time I began to have a panic attack, I would repeat that verse to myself: *God has not given ME a spirit of fear, but of power and of love and of a sound mind.* I said it over and over and over again—sometimes thirty or more times a day. It was my total focus, and I committed my heart and soul to believing it. It was easy to recall this passage, because my sense of panic seemed to haunt me at every turn. It was a constant trigger, sending me running to God's arms and his truth. Over the course of the next six to nine months, my panic attacks became much less intense, and they didn't last as long. Then they started to come less and less frequently. By the end of a year, they were completely gone and never returned.

If you have ever struggled endlessly with a destructive emotion or habit, I'm sure you can imagine the genuine joy and relief I experienced when I was fully delivered from my pain. I still thank God today for showing me the way out. And I know that if he had chosen to heal me instantaneously (as I had hoped), then I never would have learned the principles that I want to pass on to you in this book. The principles are biblical, they are powerful, and they are available to anyone who chooses to take the time to pursue God and his ways with a surrendered heart.

Don't get me wrong. Please don't think you have to be some spiritual giant to experience God's transforming power. As I already said, I was pretty ignorant about spiritual matters when God began teaching me the power of his transforming ways. And despite the many changes he has made in my mind and life, I (like everyone) am still a work in progress.

Humble Hearts Find a Powerful Place of Change

In the times when I have been the most broken, I have also been the humblest and most desperate for God. It is in this state that we are willing to surrender our will to God's and receive his instruction. In this lowly place, we cry out to our Abba Father and seek truth from his Word, and he shows us the way.

> The sacrifices of God are a broken spirit;
> a broken and contrite heart,
> O God, you will not despise.
>
> Psalm 51:17

Too often we have a plan for dealing with our issues. We go on diets, make resolutions to stop smoking, make a commitment to get our spending under control, all in our own power. We work on our behavior but not our faulty thinking. The Bible tells us in Proverbs 3:5–6 to

> trust in the LORD with all your heart
> and lean not on your own understanding;
> in all your ways acknowledge him,
> and he will make your paths straight.

We must be humble enough to acknowledge (and believe) that God has a better plan for us than any self-help guru or well-intentioned friend. He alone has the answers, and he alone fully understands who we are and what we struggle with. If this is true (and it is), why don't we immediately run to his truths and use them (and only them) to change our minds, our habits, and our lives?

> "For my thoughts are not your thoughts,
> neither are your ways my ways," declares the LORD.
> "As the heavens are higher than the earth,
> so are my ways higher than your ways
> and my thoughts than your thoughts."
>
> Isaiah 55:8–9

God's infinite wisdom supersedes anything that humans can think up for managing life. And that is why I take the time in each chapter and during our forty-day journey to show you what his Word says and how it applies specifically to the objectives of this book, which are to change your mind, change your habits, and change your life.

My Body . . . My Brain

Having spent many years as a registered nurse as well as a fitness professional, I have an obvious interest in the human body. But of all the organs of the body, I am most fascinated with the brain. And, in some profound and yet never completely understood way, the mind (that part of us that can think, experience emotions, make choices, and be conscious of self) finds its source of power from within the brain. It is all so complex . . . it simply blows my mind!

In order to pursue our first objective of changing your mind, it is helpful to understand some physiological facts about the human brain. Despite its complexity, the brain is an organ that has very specific physical needs much like any other organ. Our moment-to-moment existence requires that our brain is constantly well nourished. In fact, the brain cannot store energy. It must have a constant source of blood, oxygen, and glucose (at just the right level) to function. A variety of hormones and neurotransmitters also significantly impact how it operates. And, like any other organ, it can become diseased in various ways, from brain tumors to chemical imbalances. Medical intervention is sometimes needed when this vital organ succumbs to disease or trauma.

Sickness, Not Sin

Sometimes as Christians we refuse to see the brain in this way and therefore avoid appropriate pharmacological treatment, thinking we are weak or unspiritual when all other means have failed to deal with an issue. This is very common for those who struggle endlessly with depression. There are simply some individuals whose "wiring" or brain function is defective or more susceptible to poisons in our increasingly polluted environment (to include our food sources). We live in a fallen world and therefore struggle with bodily disease, which includes disease of the brain. If you fall into this category, you can still benefit greatly from understanding and implementing the teaching in this chapter. Yet, you may need the help of a medical doctor as well to deal with any physiological dysfunction.

Fortunately for most of us, our brain problems are mostly programming issues. We have faulty information and therefore faulty beliefs. What we need is a total mental makeover with God as our Master Designer. He's done it in my life in several areas of struggle, and he can (and will) do it in yours if you let him.

Who's in Control, Anyway?

Have you ever noticed that you often run on automatic pilot? There are routines you practice day after day, and they can influence you in many ways. For example:

You accidentally dial your best friend's phone number when you meant to call your mother. That's because you dial your friend's number more than any other.

You drive directly home when you meant to stop at the store. That's because you got distracted and simply did what you usually do, drive home.

We all make these kinds of mistakes because in our brain the most dominant message wins. That is, unless it is willfully overridden by a new message.

With the advances in medical science, we have been able to study the brain in its complexity and as a result greatly increase our understanding about how and why we think, feel, and act as we do. In the brain there are billions of neuron pathways where all our thoughts and experiences occur and are stored. Those thoughts that are experienced very frequently create physically larger neuron pathways in the brain—like superhighways. Those that are rarely experienced are like little overgrown paths.

Another exciting discovery is that the size and influence of our neuron pathways can change. If we stop thinking or doing something consistently, that particular pathway will actually start to shrink. And if we do or say something new time after time for weeks or months on end, that pathway will eventually become a new highway in our mind—a new dominant thought.

God in his wisdom designed us so that we are not easily "brainwashed" by short exposure to thoughts or experiences. Rather, it is the consistent, persistent repetition that will eventually make a dynamic change in our mind. That may be frustrating for those of us who want to change *now*. But it is a protective mechanism in God's design that also works to our advantage.

We do the things we do because we literally have been programmed to do so. So to think, feel, or act differently, we must purposely think new thoughts and take new action. Notice I didn't say to "feel new feelings." That is because, except for those intense feelings that come from an instinctive "fight or flight" response, your emotions are an outflow of your thoughts . . . or more accurately your beliefs.

If you feel worthless, it is because you believe the lie that you are worthless. And that is because you have been receiving messages (from yourself or others) that tell you that you are worthless. The same goes for anger, fear, helplessness, insecurity, and so on. You may not even know what you think or believe, but your mind has not forgotten one message. And if those messages have been played many, many times, your feelings and actions have naturally followed. Bob George says in his book *Classic Christianity*: "People are in bondage to their erroneous beliefs and it moves them into emotional and physical bondage."[1]

Old Fears Live On

One of the reasons my panic attacks were so intense was because I had battled with the fear of death since my childhood. I think two things contributed to this anxiety. First, my grandfather had a heart attack (and survived) when I was very young. It made me wonder if I too would have a heart attack, as I had no understanding of how or why they occurred, and my lack of information allowed me to have an irrational fear. I rarely shared my fears with my parents and therefore had no way to dispel them. Like many people, I had this little false belief that if I shared something, it would happen. Talk about unhealthy thinking. Some of us are actually wired with a negative volition that takes some time and effort to change once we realize it's unhealthy.

Second, despite our family's lack of faith, my mother used to say a bedtime prayer each night. I guess she just thought it was the "right thing" to do. So, she said the only one she had ever heard:

> Now I lay me down to sleep,
> I pray the Lord my soul to keep.
> If I should die before I wake,
> I pray the Lord my soul to take.

Her intentions were good, but really. . . . what kind of prayer is *that* for a child—especially one who had no idea where the Lord would take her? You know how songs and poems stick in your head like a broken record? Well, I think this one stuck in mine and influenced me for years. Repetitive messages stick, so be careful what you say to yourself and others. We can powerfully impact those we love most in negative ways without even knowing it.

Two Powerful and Transforming Changes

By using the Scripture that spoke directly to my fears over and over for months on end, my neuron pathways began to change. At first, I got some relief by simply thinking about God and the Scripture. I came to understand that I could control the intensity of the attack by simply changing my focus from my anxious thoughts to God. We can all benefit in many ways every day by intentionally refocusing on the right things.

The more powerful change came many months later when I realized that I was starting to automatically move away from my old thinking and feelings with almost no effort. It felt like a new me. It was a new me. By the end of that year, my mind had been completely renewed. Somewhere in the recesses of my brain is an overgrown, teeny, tiny neuron pathway that used to be a superhighway that led me into daily fear for five years. Today my new superhighway leads me daily to a place of peace, hope, and love. I will never clear the weeds from that old path!

The Physical Change

The first change that occurred that transformed my mind was simple physiology. The old message (or more accurately neuron pathway) shrunk, and the new message grew strong enough to replace it. I know that sounds elementary and perhaps too simple to be true. But it is truly how God designed our minds whether we believe in him or not. This principle works for every human being. That is why so many life coaches and self-help experts teach on this subject. It works. The problem is that those who don't have faith in the God who designed their brain may choose to reprogram themselves in ways that do not glorify God or fit into his perfect plan and purpose for their lives.

Many famous books such as *Think and Grow Rich* by Napoleon Hill and *Psycho-Cybernetics* by Maxwell Maltz teach excellent principles and practices to change your thinking and behaviors, and readers often experience a great outcome. Most recently, a so-called expert uncovered "The Secret" to true happiness and success and wrote a book of the same name. She attributes all feelings and circumstances in our lives to "the law of attraction," saying that the "universe" is obligated to respond in certain ways.

So, what's wrong with these kinds of approaches if they can enhance our lives in positive ways? First, some teachings are complete nonsense and totally contrary to the Word of God. Second, those that seem innocuous have one common problem: they focus exclusively on "self" without any reference to God or his purposes. If you truly want to live a dynamic, powerful, and purposeful life, you absolutely cannot do it without God. As it says in Proverbs 14:12: "There is a way that seems right to a man, but in the end it leads to death."

Many things seem good at first glance, but if they do not draw us nearer to God and help us seek him first, they actually will lead to the death of our soul. We need to be very careful about what we let enter our mind every day. Everything matters, including books, music, television, friends, and even persistent thoughts.

A couple years ago, I emerged from a difficult season that had its root in unhealthy thinking in the area of discontentment. I started to focus on the things in my life that I thought were making me unhappy. Over time, those thoughts became bigger than me. This is a great example of how we can think we are on track and become blindsided by our own unhealthy thoughts if we allow them to persist.

Of course I still loved God. I was going to church and praying. But I simply focused too long on the wrong thing until I fully believed a lie. I think this happened (in part) because I was not staying grounded fully in God's Word. I was still studying the Bible. But in truth, I was not truly surrendering to its authority and power. As I said before, a humble and contrite heart is much more receptive to God's movement.

I hope I don't disillusion you by being so transparent. But as I said before, like you, I am a work in progress. And if I've learned anything these last few years, it is that we are easily deceived—even those of us who have known and loved God for many years. Much like the story of the frog that boils to death in a pan because he never notices that the water temperature is slowly changing, we can become desensitized to our own unhealthy thinking until our minds get drawn in and contaminated by lies.

Life is painful. We live in a society that demands instant gratification. We would rather take a pill than do the hard work of changing our lifestyle. We would rather buy now and pay later. We want it all . . . and we want it all now. In this kind of culture, even Christians can be enticed by teachers who seem to understand their needs and make promises that seem to easily solve their problem. Sadly, these false teachings are sometimes even wrapped in a Christian package. The apostle Paul warned his protégé Timothy about this very thing in a letter to him.

> For the time will come when men will not put up with sound doctrine. Instead, to suit their own desires, they will gather around them a great number of teachers to say what their itching ears want to hear. They will turn their ears away from the truth and turn aside to myths.
>
> 2 Timothy 4:3–4

When the core principles that guide our lives come from the Word of God and our goals flow out of a desire to glorify God, we will realize great victory and joy. It is with that perspective that we come to understand what the psalmist meant when he wrote:

> Delight yourself in the Lord
> and he will give you the desires of your heart.
>
> Psalm 37:4

Do you see in this Scripture that our delight comes before we receive the desires of our heart? When our heart is connected to the heart of God, so are our desires. We think we know what we want and need. But we really don't. We are so influenced by the world and its values that we cannot see clearly unless we are constantly looking through the very clear lens of God's Word. That is why we fill the holes in our hearts with bad habits. In reality, the only thing that can fill those holes is God's love, which is revealed powerfully in his living Word. And, that brings me to the second and most important change that transformed my life . . . and will also transform yours.

The Spiritual Change

If I had taken a purely secular approach to changing my mind, I would have simply told myself new, healthier messages over and over until my neuron pathways changed. I'm sure I would have had good results, as many people do when they change their unhealthy self-talk. There is nothing wrong with doing that if the messages are in sync with biblical truth. But my change was more than just physical. It was also supernatural for two reasons. First, I committed my surrendered heart to God and prayed daily for him to renew my mind. When our will is aligned with God (as when we delight in him), he answers our prayers affirmatively. It says in Luke 11:9–10:

> So I say to you: Ask and it will be given to you; seek and you will find; knock and the door will be opened to you. For everyone who asks receives; he who seeks finds; and to him who knocks, the door will be opened.

In my case, the Lord answered my prayer and revealed himself to me as I began seeking him. He made it possible for me to understand and respond to the gospel of Christ. Then, he allowed me to find the Scripture that spoke directly to my heart, dispelling the lies I believed and completely renewing my mind. And even though as a new believer I had taken that passage somewhat out of context, the essence of the Scripture applied to my life—God had not given me a spirit of fear. God had given me a spirit of power and love and a sound mind, once I had received him as my Lord and Savior.

> For the word of God is living and active. Sharper than any double-edged sword, it penetrates even to dividing soul and spirit, joints and marrow; it judges the thoughts and attitudes of the heart.
>
> Hebrews 4:12

The Word of God is *living* and *active*. Take a moment to get your brain around this statement. When you open the Bible, you are not just reading a really important book. When God's Word enters the mind of a believer, it has supernatural power. My pastor, Dr. Tim Scott, taught us that the Greek word for *sword* in this Scripture is *machaira*, which is actually more like a surgical knife than a sword used in battle.

As a former labor and delivery nurse, I've scrubbed in on a lot of C-section surgeries. One thing I know about surgical knives is that they are extremely sharp. In fact, when a woman must have a repeat C-section, the old scar must first be removed. The surgical knife is so effective that it can cut right through the toughest of scar tissue with ease. Imagine if that knife was sharp on both sides. It could cut out almost anything. And that is exactly what God's Word can do in your life.

When I repeated 2 Timothy 1:7 (NKJV) over and over in my mind—"For God has not given us a spirit of fear, but of power and of love and of a sound mind"—it was like turning that double-edged surgical knife on myself. It penetrated my dark and frightened soul, cut out the lies, and replaced them with truth. That truth judged my thoughts as wrong and changed the attitude of my heart and mind. That truth completely set me free.

> To the Jews who had believed him, Jesus said, "If you hold to my teaching, you are really my disciples. Then you will know the truth, and the truth will set you free."
>
> John 8:31–32

Notice in the Scripture above that Jesus was speaking to the Jews who believed him. He tells them to *hold* to his teaching and *then* they would know the truth and it would set them free. What strikes me in this passage is that those who don't believe in Christ simply cannot have spiritual eyes to see his truth and allow it to impact their lives. Christ admonishes those who do believe to hold to his teaching in order to truly *know* the truth. It's not enough to just know something, or even just believe—we must act on that belief in order for it to completely set us free.

My pastor says, "The Holy Spirit doesn't work in a vacuum. Rather he works by animating the Word of God in our lives—making it living and active . . . renewing our minds and transforming our lives." But that can only happen when we've put it into our hearts and minds in the first place!

> All Scripture is God-breathed and is useful for teaching, rebuking, correcting and training in righteousness, so that the man of God may be thoroughly equipped for every good work.
>
> 2 Timothy 3:16–17

Hopefully by now I have convinced you of the power of the mind to respond profoundly to repeated messages or experiences. Obviously the end result—our beliefs and actions—can end up being positive or negative, good or bad, godly or ungodly. It all depends on what the mind has been fed. I pray you have fully comprehended the power of God's Word to reshape you according to his purpose and design. You can be sure when God does an extreme makeover, the results are exactly what you need.

Now It's Time to Renew *Your* Mind

Let's get practical and discuss how you can apply these important biblical principles to your own life. There are several practices that will help you begin to purposely renew your mind. We will discuss each in detail. They include:

1. Set your mind.
2. Identify the lies you believe.
3. Replace those lies with truth.
4. Practice healthy self-talk.

> For most of us, thought management is, well, un-thought of. We think much about time management, weight management, personnel management . . . but what about thought management? Shouldn't we be as concerned about managing our thoughts as we are managing anything else? Jesus was. Like a trained soldier at the gate of a city, he stood watch over his mind. He stubbornly guarded the gateway of his heart. . . . If he did, shouldn't we?[2]
>
> Max Lucado

We are just beginning the process of renewal in this chapter. Don't feel that you must go through each exercise completely right now, as we will continue to address these issues during our forty-day journey. But that being said, don't just read through these practices and assume you'll do them later. Do begin to ponder, write, and practice these things a few minutes each day as you are reading these first few chapters.

While every practice is fairly simple and easy to implement, it is the actual "doing" that will begin renewing your mind. Unfortunately, too many people never take action. Like a river, they simply follow the course of least resistance and "go with the flow," thinking their old thoughts and practicing their old behaviors. You picked up this book because you want to experience change. The first change you must make is to spend time every day on things that will renew your mind. My job is to show you how simple and time efficient it can be. Your job is to pray daily for God to give you strength and wisdom for this process and then take fifteen to twenty minutes to practice new habits of the mind.

Step One: Set Your Mind

Years ago, after a brief meeting, I invited a new acquaintance to lunch and was surprised when she answered, "Sure, I can go . . . today's an 'eating' day anyway." She went on to explain that she had "diet days" and "eat anything she wanted days." Since she'd had a donut and mocha coffee for breakfast, she declared that day an "eating" day.

Are you like that, with black-and-white or all-or-nothing attitudes that not only impact your lifestyle habits but perhaps your spiritual habits as well? Too often, we operate on automatic pilot not only in our actions but also in our attitudes. Unlike specific thoughts, attitudes influence our perspectives. Sometimes even our genetic wiring influences us toward either a positive or negative attitude, one that pursues perfection or embraces complacency. No matter what attitudes you currently hold, we are told in the Bible:

> You were taught, with regard to your former way of life, to put off your old self, which is being corrupted by its deceitful desires; *to be made new in the attitude of your minds*; and to put on the new self, created to be like God in true righteousness and holiness.
>
> Ephesians 4:22–23, emphasis added

Too often Christians have the misconception that once Christ is their Savior, he will do all the hard work of "putting off your old self." In reality, he gives us the means and the power to do so . . . and expects us to do it. One of my favorite sayings on this subject is by Oswald Chambers from his popular devotional, *My Utmost for His Highest*: "We are in danger of forgetting that we cannot do what God does, and that God will not do what we can do."[3]

Oswald also says this about our attitudes:

> Our state of mind is powerful in its effects. It can be the enemy that penetrates right into our soul and distracts our mind from

> God. There are certain attitudes we should never dare to indulge. If we do, we will find they have distracted us from faith in God. Until we get back into a quiet mood before Him, our faith is of no value, and our confidence in the flesh and in human ingenuity is what rules our lives.[4]

What attitudes do you indulge in that rule your life in negative ways? Whatever they are, God wants them to change. My first response to Ephesians 2:22–23 is to assume that this must be possible or we would not be told to do it. There must be something specific we can actually do to move in the right direction. I think we can get a clue to what that is in two other Scriptures noted below:

> Those who live according to the sinful nature have their *minds set* on what that nature desires; but those who live in accordance with the Spirit have their *minds set* on what the Spirit desires.
>
> Romans 8:5, emphasis added

> Since, then, you have been raised with Christ, *set your hearts* on things above, where Christ is seated at the right hand of God. *Set your minds* on things above, not on earthly things.
>
> Colossians 3:1–2, emphasis added

It seems clear to me that the key is to purposely "set" our minds on the things of God. This is a conscious decision to shift your thinking from your old ways to his new ways. It is the part that we can do, and God expects us to do it. Simply praying, "Oh God, please take away my bad attitudes and thoughts" is not enough. He wants you to take specific action.

Years ago I had a personalized license plate that read "IMLKNUP." It stood for "I'm looking up." It was just one of the ways I reminded myself to shift my thinking, attitudes, and perspectives. I encourage you to let your disruptive emotions and destructive habits become a trigger—not to act or feel as you always have but to remind you to immediately look up and set your mind on God's truth. At first it will feel awkward and you will sometimes forget. But the more often you do it, the sooner it will become your new default mode as you are transformed by constantly setting and resetting your mind. Yet, this is impossible if we don't have the Word of God well locked in. It is my hope that this book will help you do just that in a few key habits of your mind.

Steps Two and Three: Identify Your Lies and Replace Them with Truth

Identifying the lies you believe is extremely important to the process of renewing your mind. A good place to start is by creating two lists. The first includes all the habits or behaviors that you would like to change. As you write the lists, ask yourself this question: "What lies do I believe related to this habit?" You may not be absolutely sure what you believe. Nevertheless, write down what comes to mind.

The second list may actually help even more in identifying your actual lies. For it, you will list any negative emotions that you frequently experience that you seem to have little control over. Instead of just writing the emotions only, I would like you to write the feelings associated with those emotions.

These two steps are incomplete unless you take this exercise to the next level and identify the truths that will powerfully counteract your lies. You will see below that I have provided you a space to write and an empowering truthful statement about who you really are. There is also a place for you to write down a relevant Scripture and perhaps even turn the last two entries into your own "personal statement." Lastly, you can write or say a prayer that expresses your heart to God.

At first, completing this exercise in full may seem difficult, but with practice it gets easier; and in the human mind, "practice makes permanent"!

The actions or habits I want to change:

Overeating

The corresponding lies I believe:

Food is my comfort; I need it to feel good.

Food takes my mind off things that are bothering me.

I can't say no to the foods I love—especially chocolate and potato chips.

I can never lose weight.

The truth I will use to replace the lies:

My Scripture:

So whether you eat or drink or whatever you do, do it all for the glory of God (1 Cor. 10:31).

My personal statement:

I am in control of my food choices, and with God's help I can say no, even to my favorite foods. I never overeat. I find healthy and productive ways to take my mind off my troubles. I find constructive ways to deal with the circumstances in my life that are difficult.

My prayer:

Heavenly Father, please forgive me for being in bondage to food. I pray that you will help me to become transformed by the renewing of my mind. I desire to honor you with my body, soul, and spirit. I pray that your living Word will cut out the lies I believe and replace them with truth. In Jesus's name I pray. Amen.

The negative emotions I feel:

Shame

Frustration

Despair and lack of self-control

The corresponding lies I believe:

I am worthless because I am overweight.

I cannot control myself—I am always bingeing.

I will never change—I never stick to any new program.

The truth(s) I will use to replace them:

I am a valuable, beautiful child of God.

I can find self-control by turning to Christ.

I can do all things through Christ who gives me strength.

My Scripture:

But the fruit of the Spirit is love, joy, peace, patience, kindness, goodness, faithfulness, gentleness and self-control (Gal. 5:22–23).

My personal statement:

I have great worth because I am a child of God. My weight and habits do not define me. With God's help I am being renewed daily into his image. I am setting my mind on things above and not giving in to my lust for food. I love how I feel when I eat healthfully and do things that promote a lean, healthy body.

My prayer:

Lord, I love you so much and I ask for your forgiveness

for believing the lie that I have no self-control. Help me to walk in your Spirit so that I can experience its fruit, which includes self-control. When I am tempted, I pray that your Spirit will speak to my mind and remind me that in you I have all power to resist every temptation. I thank you that I am your child and therefore I no longer live in condemnation. I pray that you will help me walk in the power of that truth. In Jesus's precious name I pray. Amen.

Now it's your turn to begin jotting down some of your initial thoughts and feelings. You may need to use another piece of paper to continue the process. Then, when you believe you have identified some of your core issues, negative thoughts, and unhealthy emotions, begin to pray and search for Scripture that speak to your heart. Over the course of our forty-day journey, I'm sure you'll find many that will be effective in helping you renew your mind. Write these key Scriptures on index cards and keep them close at hand. I would recommend that over time you narrow it down to two or three key Scriptures. Memorize those and repeat them often. I will discuss the power of repetition in a moment. Right now, take a break from reading and please begin writing your thoughts down in the area provided below.

The actions or habits I want to change:

The corresponding lies I believe:

The truth I will use to replace the lies:

My Scripture:

My personal statement:

My prayer:

The negative emotions I feel:

The corresponding lies I believe:

The truth(s) I will use to replace them:

My Scripture:

My personal statement:

My prayer:

It may take some time to identify your lies and the specific truths and Scripture that counteract them. Remember that this is a journey. Pray daily for God to help you find those as you read each daily devotional, study the Bible, hear messages at church, or even listen to Christian radio. He is always faithful to respond to a heart that is seeking truth.

Step 4: Practice Healthy Self-Talk

Sometimes Christians get concerned when I bring up the subject of practicing "healthy self-talk." For some it sounds like a New Age practice. But it is not. In fact, the Bible speaks very specifically to what we are to think about. I think it is expressed most clearly in Philippians 4:8–9.

> Finally, brothers, whatever is true, whatever is noble, whatever is right, whatever is pure, whatever is lovely, whatever is admirable—if anything is excellent or praiseworthy—*think about such things.*
>
> emphasis added

In order to transform our minds, we must put good information into them. Over 70 percent of what we hear or read on a daily basis is negative. To counteract this we must take stewardship of our minds by purposely thinking about things that renew our minds and focus us on truth. If we don't take aggressive action, we will not only stay stuck in our current thinking, we will most likely move even further in the wrong direction. In speaking to my Christian friends, I often wonder how anyone can survive in this world without knowing Christ. How can we possibly process all the horrible things that people do and the great tragedies of life with any hope at all unless we know the whole story? And yet, even many Christians are living lives of frustration and despair. I believe that is because they are focusing on the wrong information!

The Importance of Healthy Self-Talk

While gaining truth from God's Word is the most important step toward a renewed mind, not every single thing you need to tell yourself will be found specifically in the Bible. You will need to write and say new messages that address your specific lies. Of course, these must be in agreement with biblical principles. For example, I needed to give myself some important new messages to erase and replace my old negative thoughts and feelings about food. I've listed just a few of the lies I believed below and the new "truths" I used consistently to counteract those lies:

Old message: I can't say no to tempting food.
Truth: I'm in control of my food choices and am not easily tempted.

Old message: Once I start eating, I can't stop.
Truth: I am easily satisfied and absolutely hate feeling too full. I can stop!

Old message: I can never stick to a healthy lifestyle; I always fail.
Truth: In God's strength, I can eat and live to honor him and maintain a lean, healthy body. It is a joy to eat to his glory alone.

These messages combined with many Scriptures from the Bible that speak about temptation and self-control have become resident superhighways in my mind. I cannot remember the last time that I ate too much and said, "I'm too full." I just never do that anymore. I really do hate that feeling. While I enjoy occasional "fun foods" and am not a complete purist, I never feel tempted to the point of being out of control. If you had seen how much I used to eat on my binges (enough to feed a third world country), you'd be amazed at my transformation.

Telling yourself the truth changes your mind and your behavior . . . if you do it with consistency. But don't just rely on what I have to say. I would like to share the words of a very well-respected Christian psychologist. In his book *The Healing Power of the Christian Mind*, Dr. William Backus comments on the subject of self-talk.

> As a clinical psychologist and pastor, I've been aware for decades how dark depressive thoughts and negative self-talk create more emotional problems than the actual events that trigger our emotions. Self-talk refers to the way we mentally process events—that is, how we interpret things that happen to us. That's why it's important to understand how our self-talk—those statements we make to ourselves—form our emotions: powerful feelings like fear, anger or worry.
>
> Today, I am convinced that strengthening your spirit with bold, encouraging, life-giving truths that are revealed in the Bible—God's Word—will help you move toward physical wholeness and overall well-being. The Spirit communicates with your mind and your mind communicates with your body. The truth has a positive impact on our bodies when it is believed and when it is allowed to change our state of heart—that is, our moods and character.[5]

A Simple Approach to Changing Your Thinking

Behavioral psychologist Dr. Shad Helmstetter dramatically demonstrated the principles of healthy self-talk in his own life. He had been studying the impact of how people talk to themselves in his research working with top athletes. He decided to experiment on himself and address his own challenges with losing weight.

The doctor created his own audiotape full of healthful messages about eating well and becoming more active. On the tape he told himself things such as, "I love exercise. I am in control of my eating, and I enjoy healthy foods." Each morning as he shaved at his bathroom sink, he would play his tape on a cassette player. Over the course of many months, he shed fifty-eight pounds! Interestingly, his wife, who was getting ready at the other sink, also lost weight, and it wasn't even her tape! He proved for himself the truth of how the brain is designed—the most dominant thought will ultimately drive our behavior.

Positive self-talk is something you should engage in daily. Changing your mind requires a consistent supply of powerful messages. You are personally responsible to ensure the regular delivery of those messages. If you don't choose to infuse transforming truths into your mind, you are surrendering control to your old lies or the negative influence of the world. In order for your neuron pathways to even begin changing, you must hear messages a minimum of twenty-one days. Then for those pathways to continue growing and in fact *over*grow the old messages, you must continue for many months. If you ever sense you are slipping into old mental habits, then you must go back to purposely renewing your mind with truth.

A Constant Source of Good Mental Nutrition

There is a huge difference between knowing something and truly believing it. As William Backus says, "You can identify certain foods and 'believe' they exist and in fact can nourish you, but they do not until you eat them. Like real food, truthful ideas are those that feed the soul with a healthful and true picture of reality."[6] The body and the soul need consistent nutrition to be vibrantly healthy. And once we are healthy, we don't starve ourselves once again of vital nutrients. No, we feed ourselves daily for life!

It has been my experience that people have a hard time adding new things into their already busy lives. With that in mind, I have produced healthy self-talk tapes and CDs for many years for my readers and clients. In fact, they are one of my most popular resources because they allow people to listen over and over to healthy, Scripture-filled messages while they are going about their daily routine such as driving, housecleaning, or doing other mundane tasks. Over the years I've received many letters and emails sharing how helpful this resource has been.

From Bondage to Breakthrough

When I received a phone call from Katie, a young woman who took my *Scale Down, Live It Up!* lifestyle program years before, I was surprised and delighted to learn that she had lost one hundred pounds and kept it off applying what she learned in the program. I never get tired of hearing those kinds of reports! And when I do, I want to know what things made the biggest difference in the journey. Katie explained that the reason she was calling was because one of her best tools, her self-talk tapes, were completely worn out and she wanted to order new ones. She said they had been her best source of strength as she took one day at a time and learned to renew her mind and habits. So, of course we sent her a new complimentary set (now CDs) that would last her for years to come.

At the conclusion of writing this book, I created a new *Change Your Habits, Change Your Life* self-talk CD that incorporates almost all of the Scripture and key principles in this book as well as lifestyle statements that I believe are biblically grounded and universally helpful. The CD is recorded in ten short, five- to seven-minute tracks that can be listened to as you go about your normal routine. Most people will find two or three tracks that speak especially to them. You can certainly make your own customized recording, which would also be an excellent tool for renewing your mind. If you do, be sure you speak in the first person and make all positive and uplifting comments rather than coming from a negative bent. If you would like a copy of my CD, there is more information at the back of the book.

Whether you use my CDs or your own written or recorded messages doesn't matter. What matters is that those new messages get into your brain on a daily basis. Don't underestimate how important this one exercise can be. It is so important that I have included it as one item on the daily checklist you will learn about later.

The Three Ways We Learn

It amazes me how quickly children learn. It seems like one moment they are gurgling and cooing and the next thing you know, they are crying out, "That's my toy, you can't have it!" How did they learn language so quickly? They observed, imitated, and repeated the people around them. And that's how we learn every new thing as well.

Parla Italiano?

Recently, I spent two years living in the Italian section of Switzerland in a town called Lugano, which is very near Lake Como, Italy. Since less than 20 percent of the locals speak English, I was compelled to learn Italian to simply survive. I listened to CDs for hundreds of hours, studied using many Internet language programs, and took over sixty hours of intense classroom instruction; not to mention attempting to speak with dozens of people every week. Over the course of my first year, I became decently functional in my new language. But, can you imagine the result if I had listened to someone with a Russian accent on the CDs? Or, what if I only listened to each CD once? How many phrases would become familiar enough to repeat? The few that I would learn would sound pretty funny coming out of my mouth. The reality was, I had to *observe* (mostly by listening) good role models, *imitate* them as best I could, and *repeat* those unfamiliar phrases again and again and again. Now, on occasion, after a few familiar phrases leave my mouth, a local assumes I speak fluently and rapidly fires back with a succession of sentences I can understand only partially. I have a lot more observing, imitating, and repeating to do before I move from functional to fluent. But, if I continue, I will get there! *Veramente!*

Observe

After the apostle Paul told us what to think about in Philippians 4, he went on to give us some insight on the importance of following godly role models. He says in verse 9: "Whatever you have learned or received or heard from me, or seen in me—put it into practice. And the God of peace will be with you."

Can you imagine saying something like this to someone? It is in essence saying, "Whatever I've taught you, whatever you've heard me say or seen me do, do that exact thing—and it is so good and so right—that God will be pleased and bestow great peace in your life." It is rare to find a role model in this life that can speak with such authority. But, Paul was totally sold out to God. He no longer lived for himself but for Christ who lived in him. What better role model to follow?

Unfortunately, we are often drawn to the *results* in people's lives rather than the *principles* they live by. We want to follow their processes, hoping to achieve the same in our lives. That is why we follow fad diets, seek get-rich schemes, and do all sorts of nonsensical things. The pretty supermodel on the fashion catalog may look great by many people's standards, but if we saw her real lifestyle, we would likely find unhealthy attitudes and habits keeping her thinner than most people were ever designed to be. Rather, we should first determine the principles God wants us to live by and then follow the teaching and role models that support those principles. Since we do learn by observation, imitation, and repetition—we need to get the first step right and observe the right people doing the right things.

Imitate

Second, we need to imitate the quality models we have chosen and as the Scripture above says, put into practice that which we have seen. Since God tells us to be imitators of Christ, that is the perfect place to start. Several years ago, someone came up with the clever acronym WWJD. Today most American Christians know what that stands for: What Would Jesus Do? It's a great starting place for processing every new thought or behavior. Simply pass it through a biblical grid and make sure that it honors God. And, when in doubt . . . don't!

When we first start imitating new thinking or behaviors, it feels awkward and unnatural, but over time you will become more comfortable. It is the third part of learning that is now essential to truly "own" your new thought or action.

Repeat

It is the repetition stage of change where you begin to internalize the changes desired. The longer you practice a new behavior, the easier it becomes. For many years spanning the eighties and nineties, I taught a variety of dance and exercise aerobics classes before the new "step" classes hit the scene. I was one of the first to be introduced to the new concept by its originator. I'm fairly athletic and coordinated, so I figured it would be a piece of cake . . . until I took her class. While she was moving right, I went left. She had the whole class facing the back wall, and I was facing her. What in the world happened? I simply had no neuron pathways wired for this new activity . . . and it showed! Within a few months, I was teaching step aerobics. I've learned time after time that if I take the time, I can learn (or unlearn) almost anything. Nike's slogan would be much more accurate if it said: Just do it . . . and do it . . . and do it again!

Remember what I said about your neuron pathways. They don't even begin to change for about twenty-one days. Therefore, you must exercise a certain level of personal discipline before you actually sense any internal changes that will eventually move your mental transmissions from manual to automatic.

But Wait . . . Just One More Important Thing

We've covered a lot of ground in this chapter, but there is one more important biblical truth I want to address in closing. It is my favorite Scripture on the subject, and I mentioned the first part of the verse in the introduction to this book as noted below:

> Do not conform any longer to the pattern of this world, but be transformed by the renewing of your mind.
>
> Romans 12:2

Like the Scripture from 2 Timothy that spoke to my fear, this Scripture captivated my thinking. I understood the admonishment not to conform to the pattern of the world, but I was baffled at how to practically renew my mind and experience the much-desired transformation. It is my hope that this chapter has answered that question clearly in your mind. In its simplicity, we renew our minds by filling them with God's powerful truth as much as we possibly can. This is one area of our life where we can gorge ourselves continuously and never become too full. When this transformation occurs, we experience another profound result that is expressed in the second part of the verse:

> Then you will be able to test and approve what God's will is—his good, pleasing and perfect will.
>
> Romans 12:2

When our minds are renewed and our entire being is transformed by truth, we are able to understand the will of God for our lives. His will is always good, pleasing, and perfect. But, unless you have a renewed mind, you will not be able to understand what it is and actually desire to follow it more than your old unhealthy desires.

the battle of the flesh

Years ago, my oldest daughter (now thirty-one) chose to deal with the difficulties in life by doing everything she could to numb the pain. One way she numbed it was by shopping. She spent money she didn't have and ran up incredible debt. But that didn't stop her. When she found an opportunity to make a lot of money with very little effort, she jumped on it. The problem was that trafficking drugs is both dangerous and illegal. At twenty-two years old, she was caught passing marijuana across the Mexican border and sent to a woman's detention facility for forty days. Obviously, the experience scared her to death. But forty days and a strong regret for being caught did not change her character. Without a deeply repentant heart and a commitment to renewing her mind, she simply made better choices for a while because she feared the consequences. However, over time the fear diminished. Two years later she was caught again, this time passing cocaine. The consequences were much greater—up to ten years in federal prison. Now *that* got her attention.

She did not know what her sentence would be for the first full year. In that time, she realized the outrageous price she had paid for living such an unhealthy lifestyle. She had used drugs, trafficked them, and made tons of money, but she had ultimately reaped nothing but pain. When as a parent you watch a child you love fall deeper and deeper into darkness, it absolutely rips your heart out. The hardest thing is to realize you have no control.

I had prayed for years for my daughter, sharing truth and unconditional love with her every chance I got. But, for whatever reason, she never truly responded. She had to hit rock bottom. In that prison, she came to know Christ in a personal way. She repented and started a journey of transformation that was amazing. She said to me one day, "Mom, I used to think it was so corny when you would quote Mother Teresa and say, 'You don't know Jesus is all you need until Jesus is all you've got.' Well, now I know exactly what you meant. I am so happy that God saved my life and saved my soul by allowing me to get caught." My daughter only had to spend two and a half years in prison. Today she is a beautiful young woman who has a thriving business. We are the best of friends.

Like my daughter, some of us must hit rock bottom before realizing how destructive our unhealthy habits have become. However, many of us exist just above the bottom, never in enough pain to force change, yet still wallowing in frustration and discontentment. It is my prayer that this book will be an important tool to help you conquer your flesh and move to a place of victory and freedom.

What's Your Issue?

John feels like he can't stop himself from viewing pornography on the Internet. Mary can't say no to chocolate. Bill has been smoking three packs of cigarettes a day for fifteen years. Sharon laughs when she calls herself a shopaholic, but she's not laughing inside. All these people know and love God. Yet, they feel as if they have absolutely no control when it comes to their unhealthy habits. All four are in a "battle of the flesh," and they are losing.

"Flesh" sounds so base. But that is the word the Bible uses to refer to our humanness, or how we function naturally before God gets ahold of us. It includes our body and mind and the thoughts and behaviors that flow from them. Since the fall, man has fought against his natural inclination to pursue immediate gratification. As David Needham puts it in his book *Birthright: Christian, Do You Know Who You Are?* "We dare not forget that apart from God's intervention, flesh (mortal humanness) as such, functioning independently from God, has an unavoidable bent toward sin."[1]

Before a person becomes a true believer in Christ, he or she can only follow one path of life—that of the flesh. Sometimes good and noble things are accomplished; sometimes not. But even the good things are done under human power alone and for their own gratification. It has nothing to do with God.

In the instant that you trusted Christ alone for your salvation, something miraculous took place—the Holy Spirit took permanent residence in you and made you a new person. And he is literally "jealous for you," wanting to have all of you, all of the time. And because he is constantly with you, you have supernatural power within you to say no to your flesh and to say no to sin. You have the ability to choose which path to walk: the path of the flesh or the path of the Spirit. Quite frankly, as Christians we make that decision many times (in fact, moment to moment) every single day. If you are not aware of those decisions, you are likely walking in the flesh. And the really frustrating thing is that in our "natural" state, we are actually wired to follow our flesh. This is the struggle that the apostle Paul spoke of in Romans 7:18–19 (NASB) when he wrote

> For I know that nothing good dwells in me, that is, in my flesh; for the willing is present in me, but the doing of the good is not. For the good that I want, I do not do, but I practice the very evil that I do not want.

Ever feel that way? I sure have, too many times to count . . . just yesterday! That is what happens when we follow our flesh. Fortunately, Paul did not leave us without hope. This is what he ultimately concludes with:

> Wretched man that I am! Who will set me free from the body of this death? Thanks be to God through Jesus Christ our Lord! So then, on the one hand I myself with my mind am serving the law of God, but on the other, with my flesh the law of sin.
>
> Romans 7:24–25 NASB

When we allow Christ to become Lord of our lives, it is he (through the Holy Spirit) who gives us the power to walk in the Spirit. Notice I said "allow." When we believe in Christ, he pardons us from all our sins and gives us eternal life and becomes our Savior. But, in that moment when we are miraculously saved, we are not immediately perfected. We never will be this side of heaven. But, it is God's will and our work to glorify him and allow him to transform us in the likeness of Christ while we are on this earth. When we walk in the flesh and seek our own gratification over his glorification, we cannot do that.

Plug In to the Real Source of Power

You probably own a power vacuum. Have you ever tried to vacuum your rug without plugging it in? I doubt it. You know that you need a power source to get the job done. You'd never consider vacuuming any other way. So, why do so many of us live under our own power, rather than being plugged in to the supernatural power of God? His power is always available, but we must choose to access it. I hope that this chapter will help you understand how to do just that.

Who Is the Enemy?

Beyond thinking good thoughts and meditating on God's Word, we must be filled with wisdom so we can fight the enemy and avoid the path of the flesh. In my life, I have come to realize that the enemy most often is simply me. I do a fine job on my own, going after what I think I want or need at the moment, only to regret later that I did not take a different path. But, when I am strong in the Lord and walking firm in his Spirit, I have also discovered that another enemy rears his ugly head and feeds me lies and temptations that I am not always prepared to handle. It is important that we are well equipped to fight both enemies—ourselves and Satan.

Which Path Do You Walk?

Imagine for a moment opening up your door tomorrow morning and discovering two distinctly different paths extending from your front porch, each with a sign bidding you to come. The first is breathtakingly beautiful. Its smooth stones and lush landscaping draw you in. The sign says that you must travel on your own but promises to meet every desire of your heart. You feel quite certain it will bring you immediate pleasure. The other is a much narrower path, and you cannot see beyond more than a few steps. It seems barren and rocky, with nothing compelling you to take it. But the sign says that you will have a guide who has prepared the way for you and at the end you will find great joy. Which will you choose?

The Path of Least Resistance

The first is the path of the world—the one that draws your flesh by promising to meet your immediate needs. It seems like the right choice. It feels right. Sometimes, the path of the world is simply the road you travel on your own steam. It doesn't mean that everything you do in the flesh is bad or immoral. It is simply done under your own power and for the purpose of achieving your own goals and satisfying your own desires. Those who do not know Christ can only walk this path. It still tends to be the default mode of Christians more often than not. But, it doesn't have to be that way.

The Path with Real Power

When we choose to "look up," surrender to God, and live out of love for him, this is the path of the Spirit. It is a path where both our motives and actions are pure and in sync with each other. But it's tough to stay on that selfless path; in fact, impossible under our own power. Some would have you believe that Christians can stay on the narrow path as long as they are disciplined and committed to God. This is not true. The "disciplined" walk is simply a "flesh walk" that looks spiritual. Walking with God is not a matter of discipline and commitment, it is a matter of surrender—choosing to walk in his powerful truth moment after moment.

God wants our constant thought and attention. When we learn to do this, we will always be on his perfect path. In the process, most of us will live a rather zigzagged journey as we traverse back and forth between the flesh and the Spirit. But it is a trek worth taking, despite our frequent failures, because our walk will get more and more consistent as we practice setting our minds on God.

Most of you picked up this book because you want to change your habits. If what you were already doing was working, you would not be reading this. The problem at its core is that you are walking in the flesh. Part of that has to do with your unhealthy thinking, as we already discussed. The other part is that you have not completely sold out to God in some areas of your life. In Galatians 5:16 (NASB), Paul writes: "But I say, walk by the Spirit, and you will not carry out the desire of the flesh." Now if walking by the Spirit were an automatic response to being born again, Paul wouldn't have to tell us to do it! And if it were impossible to do, he wouldn't even ask us to try. Yet he reminds us of the intensity of the struggle as he continues in verse 17 (NASB): "For the flesh sets its desire against the Spirit, and the

Spirit against the flesh; for these are in opposition to one another, so that you may not do the things that you please." It is obvious that we are in the same battle Paul had in Romans 7. All believers will battle. If they say they don't, they are lying. But they do have the power to win the battle.

In his book *Classic Christianity*, Bob George uses a powerful analogy to illustrate our ability to choose between our fleshly (often sinful) desires and the great riches we receive when we walk in the Spirit. He shares a story of a restaurant owner who finds a starving, homeless beggar digging through the dumpster behind his restaurant, looking for scraps of food. The man invites the beggar in and tells him that he can eat there every day and choose anything he wants. The beggar can scarcely believe his eyes as he looks at all the incredibly delicious food. He asks, "I can have anything?" The restaurant owner nods his head. "Yes, absolutely anything," he replies. Slowly, with a gleam in his eye, the beggar asks, "Can I still eat from your garbage bin?"[2] That is exactly what we choose to do when we choose to walk in the flesh. God has given us the liberty of choice—his riches or the world's pleasures. Why is it we so often choose the garbage?

Though this prevalent human battle of the flesh can get us frustrated, we must never give up. Paul delivers some encouraging news in Galatians 5:22–23: "But the fruit of the Spirit is love, joy, peace, patience, kindness, goodness, faithfulness, gentleness, self-control; against such things there is no law" (NASB). He says that we have crucified our flesh with its passions and desires. At first glance, it may seem as if this verse tells us that the battle is already won. But we know from his previous comments (and the evidence in our own lives) that this simply is not true. I think what he means is that our faith in Christ gives us the power to submit our self-centered worldview to a Christ-centered perspective that puts the things of God above our own fleshly desires. Notice how he continues in verse 25: "If we live by the Spirit, let us also walk by the Spirit" (NASB).

We live by the Spirit (for eternity) because we are sealed in Christ. But Paul is exhorting us to walk this earthly life consistent with our new identity. And though during this earthly walk we never completely arrive, we grow stronger and more Christlike each day if we are walking in the path of the Spirit.

Stirring Up the Spirit in Your Life

I once had a Bible teacher describe the power of the Holy Spirit in our lives using the analogy of chocolate milk. She said to imagine squirting thick chocolate syrup into a tall glass of milk. The syrup immediately sinks to the bottom of the glass. Is the chocolate in the milk? Sure. Has it permeated the entire glass of milk? No. It lies on the bottom, available but not activated. Grab a spoon and stir it up, and the whole glass of milk becomes chocolate.

This simple example illustrates how we can live with the Spirit of God *in* us without allowing him power *over* us. God could choose to override our wills at any time. He rarely does. He allows our frustration and sense of futility with our own efforts to bring us back to him eventually. Then we are forced to realize our own inadequacy and fall on our knees and ask, "How do I 'stir up' your Spirit in my life and live in your power alone, Lord?"

As I mentioned earlier, many Christians believe that leading a holy life is all about personal discipline and commitment. But we've discovered that all our human effort is still walking in the flesh, no matter how good or outwardly spiritual we are. Remember the Pharisees? They didn't impress Christ. And our human efforts don't impress him either. He doesn't want our efforts, he wants our hearts. And that is what it takes to "stir up" the Spirit and walk consistently on the path God has set before us. It takes a surrendered heart to produce the fruit of the Spirit Paul spoke about in Galatians. Consistent with Paul's teaching, John gives us a clear picture when he shares what Jesus told his disciples in the parable of the vine. Jesus says:

> Abide in Me, and I in you. As the branch cannot bear fruit of itself unless it abides in the vine, so neither can you unless you abide in Me.
>
> I am the vine, you are the branches; he who abides in Me and I in him, he bears much fruit, *for apart from Me you can do nothing.*
>
> John 15:4–5 NASB, emphasis added

Apart from Christ we can do nothing . . . that is, nothing of any real significance. So, to walk in the Spirit, to abide in Christ, we must be constantly dependent upon him. We must abide in him constantly. Abide means to stay in a given place, state, relation, or expectancy. It means to dwell, endure, remain, or stand. We all know what happens if we pull a branch off of a tree. It dies. It has no life to produce fruit. In this parable, Jesus is speaking of specific spiritual fruit—all those wonderful manifestations of walking in the Spirit Paul spoke of in Galatians—the list that ends with self-control. In fact, it appears that abiding and walking in the Spirit are the same thing. Jesus continues in John 15:7–8 (NASB):

> If you abide in Me, and My words abide in you, ask whatever you wish, and it will be done for you.
>
> My Father is glorified by this, that you bear much fruit, and so prove to be My disciples.

In the Greek, the word *abide* means to settle down and be at home. Abiding in Christ means that we are to stay close and depend on him for everything. He says that when his words abide in us, we may ask whatever we wish and it will be done. So often, we focus on the "ask whatever we wish" part of that verse and neglect the most important part—abiding. He said *when* his Word abides in us, *then* we can ask. His words cannot abide in us unless we have taken time to read, study, and meditate on them often.

Stay Close

If you are a parent or have ever cared for children, you know that they will often ask to do something they are not ready to handle. When at six years old, my daughter got her first two-wheeled bike for Christmas, she was so excited that she could barely contain herself. She wanted to jump on it immediately and ride it down the street. The problem was that she didn't know how. She didn't understand why we asked her to wait, or why we went running out to the sidewalk when we realized she had not followed our instruction. She'd seen all the other kids riding, and it looked so easy. She soon discovered after a badly scraped knee that it was a good idea to wait for Dad. With her fresh Band-Aid as a reminder of her recent accident, she willingly accepted help. As Daddy gently held on to the bike and walked beside her, she began to get her balance. She wanted him to stay very near and paid close attention to his words of instruction on how to maneuver her new bike. The sting from her fall reminded her that she should have followed his instructions the first time.

That is how it is with us every day of our lives. We need to stay very close to our heavenly Father. We need to understand his words and let them give us nourishment and life. He wants us to glorify him by bearing spiritual fruit, but there are no shortcuts. There are no blessings that come ahead of abiding. If they did, then we wouldn't abide.

What God asks of us is always possible. His methods of transformation always work. By renewing our minds and abiding in Christ moment to moment, we have the power to be all God intended. To realize this wonderful destiny requires our heart and attention. When we do this, we not only change our habits, we change our entire lives. It is amazing how foolish it is to live in our own power, following our own desires. God's path is the one with all the best rewards.

Preparing for Battle

Now that we understand the power of God working in our lives—his Word that renews our minds, and abiding that comes by daily surrender—we are equipped to face each and every temptation that comes our way.

I've often imagined how soldiers get ready for battle. Do you think that they run out onto the battlefield naked and without weapons and try to get dressed and armed in the middle of an attack? Of course not—they put on the appropriate clothes, protective vests, and helmets and then take the weapons they will need *before* they head into battle. Too often in our battle of the flesh, we walk into situation after situation completely naked and without our weapons to fight the temptations with which we've become all too familiar.

Our New Armor

In his letter to the Ephesians, Paul speaks of who we were before we knew Christ and how complete and blessed we have become now that we are his. Because we are now heirs of Christ, he tells us we are to be imitators of God as his beloved children. We are told how to have godly relationships and live in unity. In all this instruction of how to live, he concludes with these important words to prepare us for the battle of living a godly life.

> Finally, be strong in the Lord and in his mighty power. Put on the full armor of God so that you can take your stand against the devil's schemes. For our struggle is not against flesh and blood, but against the rulers, against the authorities, against the powers of this dark world and against the spiritual forces of evil in the heavenly realms.
>
> Ephesians 6:10–12

Satan wants to deceive, confuse, and distract you from being a vital Christian who not only lives in personal victory and honors God but also encourages others toward life-changing freedom in Christ. If you are stuck in bad habits and feeling defeated, he doesn't need to bother with you much. But if you are growing and glorifying God, watch out—he (or more likely one of his many agents) will be after you. Their usual method is deception that diminishes your faith. If you have not filled your mind with truth, you may believe their lies. Paul tells us how to get ready for this inevitable battle. Like a soldier going to the field, we must always be prepared.

> Therefore put on the full armor of God, so that when the day of evil comes, you may be able to stand your ground, and after you have done everything, to stand. Stand firm then, with the belt of truth buckled around your waist, with the breastplate of righteousness in place, and with your feet fitted with the readiness that comes from the gospel of peace. In addition to all this, take up the shield of faith, with which you can extinguish all the flaming arrows of the evil one. Take the helmet of salvation and the sword of the Spirit, which is the word of God. And pray in the Spirit on all occasions with all kinds of prayers and requests.
>
> Ephesians 6:13–18

It is fitting that Paul would use so many military words to describe what we must do to prepare for the enemy. When we have the full armor of God protecting us, we will always stand firm. The helmet protects our head, in this case our mind, reminding us that we are saved and complete in Christ. It is our spiritual protection from believing the enemy's lies. God's imputed righteousness and our resulting faith becomes an impenetrable shield against the enemy. The Word of God is our weapon against the lies that will be flung at us over and over as we live in this fallen world. If, on the other hand, we rarely spend time in the Word, in prayer, or in worship, we will be like naked children, vulnerable and easily captured.

Temptation

One of the areas of greatest deceit is temptation. It is where Jesus was tested. And you will be also.

> Then Jesus was led up by the Spirit into the wilderness to be tempted by the devil. And after He had fasted forty days and forty nights, He then became hungry. And the tempter came and said to Him, "If You are the Son of God, command that these stones become bread." But He answered and said, "It is written, 'MAN SHALL NOT LIVE ON BREAD ALONE, BUT ON EVERY WORD THAT PROCEEDS OUT OF THE MOUTH OF GOD.'"
>
> Matthew 4:1–4 NASB

Jesus was prepared for the battle. He had surrendered his heart and will to the Father—forty days of fasting is the ultimate submission. He had God's Word firmly rooted in his mind and heart. So, when the tempter came, Jesus, who had a great physical need for food, had supernatural spiritual strength to resist temptation. And in that moment, his "sword of the Spirit" was the Word of God.

Temptation—it's all around us. We can shop until we drop. We can eat until we pop. We can indulge our senses in every imaginable (or unimaginable) way. We see something and we want it . . . *now*. John speaks of this as the lust of the flesh, the lust of the eyes, and the boastful pride of life (1 John 2:16). Lust and pride can be so subtle that we don't even know they are present in our minds. It is easy to justify our unhealthy behavior with denial or rationalizations.

I deserve to splurge on all these decadent foods tonight. My boss has harassed me all day. I need this food to de-stress.

I can handle this magazine full of naked women. I'm not going to do anything. I'm just looking. All men do this; it's totally normal and acceptable as long as I'm faithful to my wife.

> I've had a really hard week with so many challenges. I know I'm on a tight budget, but I'm just going to window-shop and get my mind off things. I know I have a problem charging things I can't afford, but I won't let myself buy anything. I'll just look.

We tend to be tempted at our most vulnerable places. It says in James 1:14–15:

> But each one is tempted when, by his own evil desire, he is dragged away and enticed. Then, after desire has conceived, it gives birth to sin; and sin, when it is full-grown, gives birth to death.

The battle starts in our minds at the point of desire. If we don't kill the desire at its root, it is as if we are "dragged away and enticed." By that time, it is too late, and we complete the sinful act—whatever that is. It is an "evil desire" when it is something that moves us away from God and toward fulfilling anything that does not glorify him. Just as we must put on the full armor of God, we must also be careful to guard our hearts and minds from areas of temptation where we have often struggled. In 1 Corinthians 10:13–14 (NASB) we are given great encouragement by Paul in the area of our temptations. He says:

> No temptation has overtaken you but such as is common to man; and God is faithful, who will not allow you to be tempted beyond what you are able, but with the temptation will provide the way of escape also, so that you will be able to endure it. Therefore, my beloved, flee from idolatry.

Do you believe God's Word is true? I'm hoping you do and therefore fully absorb what we are taught in the Scripture above. First, you are not alone. All the temptations you experience are common. That isn't an excuse; it's simply a reality. Every human being has temptations. The most important part of this Scripture is that God will not allow you to be tempted beyond what you are able to bear. Of course you can allow yourself to be tempted despite God's provision. But, that is not God's doing. At the beginning of James 1:13, we are told that God cannot be tempted, nor does he tempt anyone. He wants to provide you with a way of escape. In fact, he's provided you with many. But, in this Scripture, the way of escape is clearly expressed: "Flee from idolatry."

In her book *Idols of the Heart*, Elyse Fitzpatrick writes: "Idolatry lies at the heart of every besetting sin we struggle with." When we are in bondage to anything—which is evidenced by repeated undesirable behavior—we are feeding our idol. Again Elyse writes: "Idolatry has to do with love—my love for God, my love for others, my love of the world." She continues, "If you are willing to sin to obtain your goal or if you sin when you don't get what you want, then your desire has taken God's place and you're functioning as an idolater."[3]

We are all guilty of idolatry at times. And we are commanded to flee. It is our best means of escape. In that moment when a thought about your "idol" comes to mind, flee. At the first sign of temptation, flee. When you think it is too late and you are already engaged in the temptation, flee.

I have noticed that many Christians seem to expect that God will provide some kind of miraculous deliverance from every temptation. They expect the phone to ring and call them away from the cookie jar. I don't think so. Who exactly is forcing the cookie down their throats? I'm sorry to be so blunt, but in all my years of compulsive bingeing, not one cookie jumped into my mouth without my help! God gives you the way of escape out of every temptation. Will you stay or will you flee?

And as you flee, pray to the one who can sympathize with your weakness.

> For we do not have a high priest who is unable to sympathize with our weaknesses, but we have one who has been tempted in every way, just as we are—yet was without sin. Let us then approach the

> throne of grace with confidence, so that we may receive mercy and find grace to help us in our time of need.
>
> Hebrews 4:15–16

Too often in shame and guilt, we run from God rather than to him. Perhaps we think he is finally disgusted with us. But he isn't. When you turn from your flesh and pursue him, he is waiting with open arms to give you mercy and grace in your time of need. He doesn't condemn and reject you. He embraces you. That is one reason why this forty-day journey is so important. You need to run to Christ every day to find your strength. Make it your new, healthy habit. Approach him in reverence and love . . . but also with confidence. He wants you to overcome. He is your "overcomer." As it says in James 4:10: "Humble yourselves before the Lord, and he will lift you up."

We will address this subject of temptation and the battle of the flesh again during our forty days. In closing this chapter, I encourage you to make the words of Paul below a prayer as you let the Lord guide you over every mountain and through every valley of this life on our way to our ultimate destination.

> That He would grant you, according to the riches of His glory, to be strengthened with might through His Spirit in the inner man, that Christ may dwell in your hearts through faith; that you, being rooted and grounded in love, may be able to comprehend with all the saints what is the width and length and depth and height—to know the love of Christ which passes knowledge; that you may be filled with all the fullness of God.
>
> Ephesians 3:16–19 NASB

4

change your habits

The restaurant was one of the best in San Diego. The menu was expansive with so many wonderful choices. But that wasn't why I couldn't seem to make a decision. It had been hours since lunch, but for some reason I wasn't particularly hungry. Nothing appealed to me at that very moment. I ordered an appetizer and salad just to be polite and marveled at the new woman who said no to a five-course meal simply "because." Now, don't get me wrong. I still love food. It's just that I don't love it all the time. I'm easily satisfied and rarely feel like eating unless I'm hungry. I can't tell you how liberating it is to be at this point. Twenty-five years ago, the thought of staying lean for decades and being released from bondage to my food obsession seemed impossible. I'm here to tell you that it is not. It is also possible for you to have the same kind of victory in your life.

Fast-Forward

Imagine for a moment that one year from today all the bad thinking and bad habits you've struggled with for so long are absolutely gone! Envision how it feels to be out of bondage and at peak health and vitality. You are content and full of joy. Each day is an exciting adventure. That can be a reality for you if you will stay on this journey until the end. And when you are done, it will be important to review and revisit the principles and practices until you know for certain they are permanently locked in. I encourage you to read the previous chapters several times and to go through the forty-day journey periodically until you know your new habits are permanently locked in.

All we've discussed thus far—renewing our minds and fighting the battle of the flesh—are vital things that must be practiced regularly to realize God-honoring change. But we must also begin to address our actual lifestyle habits. By that I mean the way you live in your physical dimension day after day. Some of these habits are necessities, like eating and sleeping. Others may include activities such as smoking, excessive shopping, or living an extremely sedentary life. It is not the intention of this book to give in-depth advice on every type of unhealthy habit. Rather, I would like to point out the obvious—what a healthy lifestyle really looks like. In this chapter we will briefly address the following lifestyle areas:

nutrition and fat management
activity and exercise
rest and regeneration
destructive lifestyle habits

I have covered the first two items in great detail in my previous book, *Scale Down: A Realistic Guide to Balancing Body, Soul & Spirit*. If you want in-depth teaching about these topics, I highly recommend you read *Scale Down* at some point. In it I address the number one unhealthy habit that plagues over 65 percent of all Americans—overeating. And though I discuss the mental and spiritual dimensions in *Scale Down*, I sensed God was prompting me to go deeper and to give more specific direction in these critical areas.

Back to Basics

There is so much information available about what it means to lead a healthy lifestyle that some people are totally confused and others are exasperated. If it was truly difficult to live healthfully, God would have created us with a user manual. We need to think back to how people lived a few centuries ago and realize that we don't need a doctorate in nutrition or physiology to find the answers. Nevertheless, I will cover some lifestyle basics in this chapter.

The truth is that most people know *what* to do when it comes to living a healthy lifestyle; they just don't know *how* to do it. As we take a look at the first three lifestyle categories above, I will simply point out what many of you will think is obvious. (It never hurts to be reminded of the things we know but don't always practice.) For example, to lose weight you need to eat fewer calories than you burn. (It really is that simple.) You also know that you need to eat lots of fruits, vegetables, and other whole natural foods. Yet, most of us fail to eat in ways that fuel our bodies sufficiently to meet all its changing demands. Like a good personal trainer (who sometimes repeats herself), I'll gently remind you to get back to basics.

In addition to the simple principles outlined in this chapter, I will include a section in your daily readings called "Nourish Your Body" that will give you greater insights and motivations to treat your body with greater respect and care. It is my intention to help you virtually see the inner workings of your body in a way that will motivate (and perhaps scare you) into caring for it more effectively.

Beyond the Average Lifestyle Challenge

If you picked up this book because you are struggling with habits or addictions that far surpass the usual lifestyle issues, I will also briefly address those in general terms. I am not a psychologist or licensed counselor. So, my advice will be fairly simple. God can work powerfully in the life of a believer who is totally surrendered. Perhaps like me you will find total renewal and victory without seeking professional help. But that being said, I do believe that God uses qualified Christian psychologists, therapists, and counselors to help you walk the road to complete recovery. Do not hesitate to seek godly counsel if you need it. In fact, I encourage you to do so.

No matter what your key issue, it may be helpful to at least skim the entire chapter, even if you think you are doing fine in some categories. One exception: if you are one of those rare people who have never struggled with your weight, skip the section on fat management. Most of us can find ways to slightly improve our nutrition, activity level, or ability to de-stress. I know that I'm still a work in progress. Each year I notch up my lifestyle in new ways. Now in my midfifties, I am more motivated than ever to maintain a reasonably youthful, lean, and fit body for whatever years the Lord has left in store for me.

How Do You Really Feel?

Think back to the last time you felt really awful. For some of you, it's hard to remember the last time you felt really good. Our health and how we feel physically impacts every aspect of our life. When we are ill, exhausted, or completely out of shape, it's hard to celebrate life to the fullest. How can we be all God intended us to be when we are falling apart? We can't. Your body is your one and only vehicle for life. It can't be traded in. So, it makes sense to care for it.

Ferrari, Bentley, or Rolls Royce, Anyone?

Imagine if a very wealthy friend gave you his extremely expensive and beautiful car to drive for a year while he was out of the country. He told you to enjoy it like it was your own but to take good care of it. What great fun. What great responsibility. As you enjoyed the power and luxury of his car, I'm guessing you would also be a little worried that you might damage it in some way. So, you would keep it filled with exactly the right fuel, get the oil changed when needed, and most likely store it in a garage when you were not driving it. Funny, many of us don't give that kind of attention to our bodies, which are really on loan from God.

> Do you not know that your body is a temple of the Holy Spirit, who is in you, whom you have received from God? You are not your own; you were bought at a price. Therefore honor God with your body.
>
> 1 Corinthians 6:19–20

How do we honor God with our bodies? First, we take good care of them by eating the right foods in the right amounts and getting adequate exercise and sufficient rest. Second, we use them as God intended, staying pure sexually and using them to carry out good deeds that show love to others and honor God. I share this important perspective because we need to get our hearts around the fact that God cares about how we live physically. If you are chronically overweight or damaging your body (be it ever so slowly) by poor lifestyle habits, you are dishonoring God. Changing your lifestyle is not just about achieving a healthier or leaner body; it is more importantly about glorifying God.

So does that mean we can never eat cheesecake or that we must become fitness fanatics? No, of course not. We don't need to over-spiritualize every little action. God gave us our incredible senses to enjoy life. I think we can have a piece of cheesecake and thank God for our sense of taste. The problem comes when we indulge ourselves (with food or anything else) to excess and reap the negative results. In the Bible there were times of feasting and times of fasting. But more often, there was day-to-day moderation. People had to sleep because there was limited light at night. People had to move because they had no other option. People ate what was available when they were hungry, if they were blessed enough to have sufficient food. Only the very rich had the luxury to become fat. With simplicity and moderation as our mind-set, let's look at the essentials of a healthy lifestyle, starting with our nutritional needs.

Nutrition

> Then God said, "I give you every seed-bearing plant on the face of the whole earth and every tree that has fruit with seed in it. They will be yours for food."
>
> Genesis 1:29–30

> Everything that lives and moves will be food for you. Just as I gave you the green plants, I now give you everything.
>
> Genesis 9:3

Nutrition for Maximum Energy

It sounds cliché, but you really are what you eat. God has created our bodies with perfect blueprints and programs to make new cells in every part of the body. It is our job to give our bodies the building materials to generate high-quality replacement parts. Skin and blood cells regenerate very quickly and our skeletal system very slowly. But, within seven years every single cell in your body will be different than what you have at this very moment. (And that is a profound spiritual thought in itself.) My question to you is this: of what quality will that new body be? It will depend on the foods you eat (or don't eat) every single day. If you simply improve the quality of your nutrition 10 to 20 percent in the next year, your body will respond in remarkable ways.

> When God created humans, He also provided all the nutrients we needed to maintain a healthy body. He did not hide those nutrients

> from us, and He didn't package them separately and write a book to explain exactly how each one functions. He simply put an abundance of nutrients in the foods that we would eat.[1]
>
> Dr. James Balch

Eating to build the best new body possible is not really very complicated. For most of us, it means decreasing the empty calories and adding more nutrient-dense foods to our daily diet. With that in mind, I've created five simple nutritional principles that can help you increase your energy and build healthy new cells every day. As I already said, you know most of this information. As you read, ask yourself, *Am I implementing these principles consistently?*

Habit #1: Water

Your body must have a constant supply of water to survive. Most people die of dehydration within a few days without it. Your body doesn't sweat soda or iced tea, it sweats water and electrolytes. It needs water to perform all of its bodily functions, and when you don't drink enough, it resorts to handling only the most essential functions. Many people live with chronic low-grade dehydration resulting in a variety of negative outcomes such as low energy, poor skin tone, and inadequate fat metabolism, to name a few. Try to drink at least four to eight ounces of water for every hour you are awake. If you wait to drink it until you're thirsty, you're already at least a quart low. If you want to look younger, have more energy, and live longer, drink pure, fresh water all day long. This is an essential habit for good health.

Habit #2: Lots and Lots of Plant Foods

Fiber-rich fruits, vegetables, whole grains, beans, legumes, seeds, and nuts are packed with vitamins, minerals, phytochemicals, antioxidants, and fiber that help fight cancer, provide antiaging protection, and more. Study after study shows increasing evidence that this area of nutrition will have the most profound long-term effect on your health and vitality.

Supplements cannot completely fill in the gaps left from not eating enough whole foods. In plant foods, the fiber alone has an incredible balancing effect on blood sugar. By eating at least five to ten grams of fiber-rich foods at every meal, you will stay full longer and have higher energy. High fiber also greatly benefits your entire digestive system. And don't forget that your breads and cereals should have enough whole grains to be considered a complete food. Look for at least three to six grams of fiber in cereals and two to four grams in breads. Most refined, packaged foods enter the body and are turned to sugar and paste within minutes of ingestion. No wonder we feel so sluggish after eating too many empty calories.

Another important reason to increase your plant food intake is to bring your body back into the right acid/alkaline balance. When we ingest too much acid from foods like protein, sugar, coffee, and carbonated beverages, our bodies become inflamed and more susceptible to illness. Only plant foods can counteract this acid and diminish those ill effects. The problem is that the American diet is extremely low in this area. When we are balanced, our energy increases, it is easier to lose weight, and our overall health soars. I will teach more extensively on this subject in one of the "nourish your body" segments during your forty-day journey.

Habit #3: Quality Protein

Protein is essential for tissue repair and maintenance and for the growth of muscles, blood, hormones, enzymes, and antibodies. You should always eat some protein with breakfast and lunch, because like fiber, it digests very slowly and stabilizes your blood sugar. A stable blood sugar promotes higher energy and diminishes hunger. However, more is not always better. Too much protein can overtax your body, particularly wreaking havoc on your kidneys. There is absolutely no healthful evidence to validate the outrageous propensity toward high-protein diets. Why did God create such an incredible array of colorful foods for us to eat if we were designed to be predominately carnivores? For now, try to get at least twelve to fourteen grams of protein at both breakfast and lunch. Also, find creative ways to add a little protein to your snacks, such as nuts or peanut butter on whole grain crackers. Protein at dinner is not as important as earlier in the day. I know this runs contrary to American customs, but at the very least, we would do well to eat at least half our usual portion in the evening.

Habit #4: Healthy Fats

Choosing the right fats and understanding their benefits and drawbacks will help you dramatically in your weight management efforts. Keeping the right amount of healthy fat in your diet will leave you feeling full and satiated longer than a nonfat meal. Fats have long been getting a bad rap, but the truth is that some are essential to your health. The key is to eat the right kind because, as with carbohydrates, not all are created equal. Lots of people simply eat too much fat. But many more get almost none of the vitally essential omega-3 fatty acids that have a crucial impact on our health. This essential fat dramatically impacts brain function and cardiac health and has been linked to positive protection from Alzheimer's disease. It is also an incredible beauty aid as it provides the vital nutrients to promote healthy skin.

For now, try to reduce the saturated (animal and dairy) fats as much as possible. The total fat in your diet should range between 15 and 30 percent. Stay on the lower end until you reach your ideal size. Olive oil is always a good choice for cooking and salads. Or try adding omega-3 fats to your diet by eating cold-water fish like salmon and tuna at least two times per week. Walnuts and flaxseed are also very high in omega-3 fat.

Unfortunately, due to pollution, heavy metals like mercury have contaminated fish all over the world. Salmon is actually the only food that can give you an adequate supply of omega-3 nutrition in one six-ounce serving. But if you eat salmon every day, you'll glow in the dark. The sad reality is that we must all supplement daily to get enough vital omega-3 fats. I have been taking an omega-3 supplement called Coromega for about five years, and my skin is better than it was in my forties. If that's not motivation enough, I know I'm going to have a healthier brain as I replace all my worn-out gray-matter cells day after day.

Habit #5: Vitamins, Minerals, and Supplements

Vitamins and minerals are nutrients that occur naturally in foods and are essential for health yet provide no calories. Antioxidants are a specific group of nutrients that form an army to capture the metabolic waste products called free radicals and transport them out of the body before they can damage the cells. All these micronutrients act like spark plugs, working to help the body do its various functions effectively. They also help us more effectively utilize our food as fuel and prevent nutritional deficiencies.

> Many of our foods have become so processed, preserved and full of chemicals that they are hardly foods at all, but rather manufactured products that happen to be somewhat digestible.[2]
> ~ Dr. Francisco Contreras

God provides all the nutrients we need in natural foods. The problem is that we don't eat the amount and variety of whole foods necessary to meet all our nutritional needs. We also have corrupted our natural food sources with depleted soil, polluted water, and chemical agents like pesticides. Today it's important to take vitamins and minerals as an insurance policy. However, they do not take the place of healthy eating. New spark plugs won't make your car run better if you forget to put gasoline in your car. And vitamins without good food are of little value.

If you're not already taking vitamins, start with a good multivitamin mineral complex and an antioxidant formula. Then, if you have a specific need, supplement based on the recommendations of your health-care professional. A word of wisdom: don't spend a fortune on micromanaging your nutrition before you get the basics down. Taking supplements will not take the place of habits 1–4 above. I have included a list of the top ten most important supplements in one of the "Nourish Your Body" segments.

Pick Your Poisons

If you could see the direct impact that some foods have on the cells of your body and realize the negative potential, you'd probably eat them anyway. Why? Because they taste so good. Most of us feel like we're being punished if we don't indulge our taste buds with our favorite foods. But when we do this on a daily basis, our body responds with excess weight, decreased immunity, increased disease, and low energy. You'd think we'd care more. But immediate, delectable gratification is a pesky little devil.

If someone told you that there was arsenic in the plate of brownies on the table, you'd definitely avoid them. But, if it was just a teeny little bit that wouldn't make you feel sick or die, and these brownies were the only chocolate dessert on the planet . . . you might just consider a bite. In essence, we are slowly poisoning ourselves by constantly indulging in empty calorie foods that are robbing us of our health and vitality. Don't get me wrong. I'm far from a purist. I do enjoy a small ration of empty calories, but I have learned the value of consistent moderation and reaped the greater reward.

Enjoying a food just because it tastes good can be done in moderation if we don't overrationalize what moderation really is. Each year that I research and teach about this topic, I have a harder and harder time indulging with joy. I simply cannot eat some things with reckless abandon anymore. Not because they are fattening but because they are unhealthy. All the facts just keep ricocheting off the walls of my brain and tormenting me if I start to go overboard. That may seem like a foreign concept to some of you, but it is a great freedom to move from craving foods that have no value to having little or no interest in them.

I actually ate a donut the other day—my first in years. It is my personal rule to save any empty "fun food" choices until after lunch if I'm going to allow myself to indulge. The donut tasted great. But all morning long . . . as my energy hit the floor, I kept thinking, *It didn't taste good enough to feel this tired an hour later.* It was a good reminder of why I don't make that choice very often. There are just a couple things I have a hard time saying no to, like pumpkin pie and my mom's homemade Christmas cookies. I let those fall into my "feasting category" and truly celebrate and enjoy every bite. But because of my years of healthy self-talk, I'm easily satisfied without feeling legalistic or superrestrictive. If someone serves dessert, I will eat a portion of it. If a friend wants to share a slice of pie, I might eat a third of it. Because I know that I can have anything I want, anytime I want it, I rarely crave it. I crave a healthy, high-energy body more.

I share all this to illustrate how seeing each bite you take for what it really is can change your attraction to it if you force yourself to acknowledge truth each time you are eating it. By deciding to think differently about the foods that can do you harm, you don't feel so compelled to eat them. With all this in mind, I'd like to give you a few motivating facts about several hazardous ingredients found in many of our favorite indulgences.

Hazardous Substance #1: Sugar

Sugar tastes good to your taste buds and acts badly in your body. It simply is not good for you. Sucrose, fructose, lactose, raw, confectioners, or "natural" sugar may have some minor differences but ultimately metabolize similarly in your body. Though your brain needs a constant supply of glucose (blood sugar) to survive, it doesn't need it in such a simple form. Our bodies are great at converting any kind of food to glucose in order to provide an ample supply to our brains. Excess sugar reacts with proteins in the body and produces a damaging effect similar to free radicals. It promotes aging, decreases your immunity, promotes weight gain, and increases your incidence of diseases like diabetes.

Refined sugar has only been part of our diets since the mid-1700s. Today, the average American consumes about two to three pounds of it each week. We've become a country that loves convenience, but all those bags, cans, and packages of processed foods are dense with sugar. While a sugar-free diet would be ideal, we don't have to throw all sweet foods out of our lives forever. But we do need to cut back our weekly intake significantly from pounds of sugar to ounces. I follow a couple of personal rules that I think work very well. As I mentioned, I almost never have anything sweet before lunch. I rarely drink beverages with sugar or fructose, and I keep my desserts or other sweet selections to no more than two hundred to three hundred calories per day. But that doesn't mean I have them every single day.

Hazardous Substance #2: White Flour

Refined bread products, white-flour pastas, crackers, and the like convert very quickly to sugar. In fact, if you put a piece of white bread in your mouth for a few minutes, you will notice a sweet taste. The starch is converting to glucose. Yes, your white bread is fortified with important vitamins and minerals, such as iron and folic acid, and contains a smidgen of protein and fiber. But for the most part, refined carbohydrates are sweet nothings. Think of it this way: every slice of white bread you eat is a bit like eating three or four vitamin-fortified marshmallows. A cup of pasta equals eight marshmallows.

Have you ever mixed a little water into a big bowl of white flour? What do you get? Paste! And that is what too many crackers and other processed foods are becoming in your digestive tract. It may sound extreme, but I label French bread, white bagels, and most crackers right up there with other junk food like chips, cookies, and cakes.

If you're not doing so already, read labels carefully and look for products that say whole grain and include two to four grams of fiber (or more) per serving. When you do choose to indulge in something sweet, a little fiber will actually slow the release of the sugar and help stabilize your blood sugar. Fortunately in recent years there are many good companies and markets offering healthier alternatives without sacrificing taste. You may not love every new product you try, but you'll probably discover a few that will become favorites.

Hazardous Substance #3: Bad Fat

If you were to get your blood drawn right after a fatty meal, you would be horrified. Sometimes you can actually see the fat in the tube of blood as it comes out of your vein! I wish that God had given us personal scopes to see what was happening microscopically inside our bodies moment to moment. I truly believe it would motivate us to stop doing some things and start doing others.

The point is that most of us are eating way too much saturated and trans fat. All those years we were eating margarine and thinking we were doing the right thing, we were actually deceiving ourselves. As it turns out, when vegetable oil is hydrogenated to be solid at room temperature, it produces trans fats that act much like saturated fats. The problem is that we are getting unhealthy fat from a multitude of sources. The obvious source is meat and dairy products. But much of the fat is hidden in our packaged foods. Become a "fat detective" and start getting some of that sludge out of your diet today!

Hazardous Substance #4: Artificial Sweeteners

Saving calories any way we can sounds like a noble quest. Yet, using artificial sweeteners on a regular basis sets you up for some possible health issues that could easily be avoided. While sugar and white flour are empty calories that create problems when taken in excess, artificial sweeteners are chemicals (despite their "natural" origins) that your body cannot always effectively expel from your body.

The most widely known artificial sweeteners are aspartame and saccharin. You'll find these in diet foods like frozen desserts, soft drinks, chewing gum, gelatin, no-sugar-added baked goods, and tabletop sweeteners. Many studies are showing that these products actually increase our sugar cravings. A study done at Harvard and other medical centers in the Boston area in the 1980s found that eating saccharin was the single most reliable predictor of weight gain. Despite sugar's downside, most nutritionists recommend using a small amount of it over artificial products.

Saccharin (Sweet'n Low) is 350 times sweeter than sugar. Studies show that it can cause cancer of the bladder, uterus, ovaries, skin, blood vessels, and other organs. Some experts state that it appears to increase the potency of other cancer-causing chemicals.

Aspartame (Equal) has generated more FDA complaints than any other additive on the market. There are actually three rooms full of boxes of complaints for this sweetener alone. Aspartame crosses the blood-brain barrier, an extremely important filter protecting the brain from contamination. This means aspartame can get directly into our brains. People who use it have reported a variety of symptoms including dizziness, hallucinations, headaches, forgetfulness, fatigue, and the like. The bottom line is that you are putting your health at risk if you use this product regularly.

Splenda entered the market in 2003 and gained quick popularity. Splenda is converted from cane sugar to a no-calorie sweetener. It isn't recognized as sugar by the body and therefore is not metabolized. While promoted as a "healthful" and "natural" product since it is derived from sugar, its chemical structure is very different from that of sugar and is actually a chemical substance.

Dr. Joseph Mercola, author of *Take Control of Your Health*, says this about Splenda:

> It is important to recognize that Splenda is basically chlorinated table sugar and as such, may have many of the risks of chlorine. It is important to recognize that it is not the safe chemical it is being promoted as. I would advise caution as many have started to report

adverse reactions to it. Splenda bears more chemical similarity to DDT than it does to sugar. Are you willing to bet your health on this data? Remember that fat soluble substances, such as DDT, can remain in your fat for decades and devastate your health.[3]

The Good News

There are a few healthful, noncaloric alternatives available. Like artificial sweeteners, they have their own unique taste that varies slightly from the sugar or favorite "sweet poison" you are familiar with, but you can acquire a taste for a healthy alternative over time if you give it a chance.

Stevia is a natural sweetener made from chrysanthemums that has almost no calories and no known side effects or dangers. At present, it can be purchased in health food stores as a sweetener, but it is not currently released to be used as an additive in foods. This is my sweetener of choice for tea and it also has a slight alkalizing effect, which most of us need.

Xylitol is a sweetener that occurs naturally. It can be found, for instance, in berries, fruit, vegetables, and mushrooms. It is safe and can be found in most health food stores.

Lo Han is a natural alternative to sugar that is safe, healthy, and can be used in a variety of ways. You can cook with it, bake with it, or mix it with tea and coffee. One serving of Liquid Lo Han Sweetener equals approximately twenty-four grams of sugar in sweetness. It has a slight molasses taste and like the others can be found in health food stores or on many websites.

Fat Management

> All man's efforts are for his mouth, yet his appetite is never satisfied.
>
> Ecclesiastes 6:7

Scale Down without the Scale

The scale was my enemy. It told me if I was fat or thin (usually fat), and if my behavior had been good or bad (usually bad). At least that's what I believed in my twenties. In reality, on a day-to-day basis, the scale doesn't tell you how fat you are or how healthy your lifestyle is. It only tells you what you weigh. If you retain extra water for some reason, you may weigh three pounds more than you did yesterday. If you are down two pounds, you may think that you're doing something right; maybe you did—or maybe you're simply dehydrated.

I don't address the subject of weight management in my teaching because weight is not the primary issue. Weigh yourself right now, then drink sixteen ounces of water and see how much you weigh. You already know what the answer is—you'll weigh a pound more. That's how easy it is to shift your weight on the scale. Weighing once a month will give you a sense of how much fat you are gaining or losing. But daily or weekly weigh-ins can be very deceptive and often discouraging. You don't need a scale to tell you how you are doing day to day if you are doing the right things. It is only one tool in determining your progress. Use it wisely. If you consistently follow the principles of good nutrition and energy balance, you will lose body fat.

I have a few statements that I've shared with thousands of people over the years that I believe are grounded perspectives for a healthy lifestyle and effective fat management. They are:

You must lose fat the same way you plan to keep it off—with a new and realistic lifestyle.

Ask yourself this question: can I eat, exercise, and live this way most days for the rest of my life and actually enjoy my life? If the answer is yes, you've found a realistic lifestyle. If the answer is no, you are probably on another diet!

Do the right things for the right reasons and trust God with the results.

As I've already said, I am not going to teach every detail about fat management in this chapter. But, I think you'll find that you'll receive more than enough information on these pages to get you on the right track. Most people don't need tons of details anyway. They just need to consistently follow a few key principles. Whether you are ten, twenty, or one hundred plus pounds overweight, these principles and recommendations can be effective . . . if you follow them *consistently*.

God versus Dr. Atkins

There are many fad diets these days that include the high protein, low carbohydrate craze of the last ten years. Do you think that God forgot to consult Dr. Atkins when he created the banana? God created quality carbohydrates, fats, and proteins as a source of fuel for human beings. In the Old Testament he also gave a few dietary restrictions, which actually still make a lot of sense. I recommend that you read my friend Jordan Rubin's book, *The Maker's Diet*, if you want to fine-tune your diet to the max. But, for our purposes, I simply want you to use your common sense to eat toward the goal of achieving excellent health and a reasonably lean body. With the previous nutritional basics already discussed in mind, let's explore the reality of how and why your body burns fat most effectively.

Four Fat-Burning Factors

Boosting and sustaining a strong metabolism is influenced by several physiological factors:

1. Gender
2. Genetics
3. Nutrition
4. Exercise/muscle maintenance

Gender and genetics are out of your control, but the other two factors are completely up to you. The principles of fat metabolism hold true despite your genetics, health, and diet history. If you are not a "fast burner," it may take longer to lose weight and you may not get the ultimate results you hope for, but you will move in a positive direction toward a reasonably lean body. Often those who struggle the most are the very ones who have damaged their natural ability to burn fat because of chronic dieting. If we follow some basic principles, we can all move in a positive direction, despite our past choices. Many health experts agree that only about 30 percent of our health (including weight) is impacted by things out of our control. Fortunately, about 70 percent is directly within our own power of choice. Those are called lifestyle choices.

The Bottom Line to Your Bottom Line

While all four factors will influence your ability to burn off excess fat, the bottom line in losing excess weight is simply "calories in versus calories out." I know that doesn't sound very sexy, but it's true. Your body is an energy bank. It stores and releases energy based on deposits and withdrawals. Most of us are making too many deposits and not enough withdrawals. Our body is a perfect calorie-counting machine. It is absolutely accurate. When someone says, "I don't know what went wrong; I gained twenty pounds over the last year!" I can tell you exactly what went wrong. The person ate more calories than he or she burned.

Here's a Pretty Amazing Little Fact

If you eat ten calories more each day than you burn, you will gain ten excess pounds in ten years. That's right . . . ten calories . . . two breath mints. The good news is that the reverse is true as well. But who wants to take ten years to lose ten pounds? My point is that small changes can make a big difference when they are practiced consistently. So as you read the information below about burning fat, don't allow yourself to get overwhelmed by all the facts and numbers. Just do something that moves you in a positive direction. Each day you can take another little step and apply more and more of what you know.

Here's a Really Simple Change That Could Work for You

It is my theory that most people who struggle with excess fat storage take in most of their calories in the last six hours of the day. If those people would simply cut their calories in half the six hours before going to bed, they would burn off significant adipose reserves. Since I can't really test my theory, why don't you test it on yourself and see how it works. Give it six weeks and then send me an email. We'll start a "Lean Evenings" club.

Keeping Things Simple with Portion Control

For those of you who freeze up when facts, data, and numbers are mentioned, I've got a solution for you. If you want to keep things really simple when it comes to counting calories, try reducing your portions by at least a third or more on almost everything you eat. The exception: fruits and vegetables. Eat more of those, not less! If you make this a consistent practice (at least 75 percent of the time), it will work. Now, here come the numbers in the next paragraph. Come on . . . give it a go. It's time to learn what your body already knows!

How Many Calories Do You Burn?

The average American woman burns about 1,700 calories per day. (The average man burns about 2,300.) At the turn of the century, she probably burned closer to 2,500 per day. That's a huge difference. Why? In earlier days, our lifestyles were much more physically demanding. Today, our automated, sedentary lifestyles dramatically minimize our calorie burn, often by five hundred to a thousand calories per day. We need to move and exercise purposefully to get that kind of calorie burn. Most people are not moving enough to stay healthy, let alone burn all the calories they eat.

My Energy Equation

For almost a decade, I've used a little device called the Caltrac Activity Monitor that tells me how many calories I burn all day long. Based on my age, height, weight, and sex, it calculates my resting metabolic rate (the number of calories I burn lying flat for twenty-four hours) and my moving calories (the number I burn in my daily activities). I learned that I burn almost 1,400 calories lying flat doing absolutely nothing for twenty-four hours. (No, I didn't just lie there—the Caltrac did!)

If I go through my normal day without any purposeful activity, I burn another 200 to 300 calories, for a total of about 1,700 calories in 24 hours. But, I came to realize that my appetite is satisfied with about 2,000 calories per day. So if I eat 2,000, and only burn 1,700 calories, those extra 300 calories are being stored as fat on my body. Obviously to maintain my weight, I must eat less or move more. I choose to move more. By adding another 300 calories of activity to my day, I am more fit and energetic and never feel like I'm on a diet. When I can't get that much activity, then I eat less. Caltrac is like my activity coach that keeps me motivated to move more every day—a benefit no matter how much you weigh.

Time to Do a Little Math Again

There are 3,500 calories in one pound of fat. So if you burn 500 calories more than you eat every day, you will lose one pound of fat each week (7 days × 500 = 3,500). That being said, in the first few weeks of a "diet," your weight on the scale seems to drop significantly, giving you great encouragement and motivation. That is because the change in your eating and the drop in your excessive carbohydrate stores cause your body to release a lot of excess water. As you continue with your new lifestyle, this will decrease dramatically even though you are doing the same thing. And as a result, you may become discouraged. This is why I must repeat: if you must weigh yourself, do so only once per month. If you consistently burn 500 calories per day more than you eat, you will melt excess fat off your body. The scale may not show the first two pounds, but I guarantee you will see and feel it. Trust the process and don't let the scale be your only measure of success. If you need to measure, use a tape measure, which is far more accurate.

Work Both Sides of the Equation

I recommend a combination of increasing output (calories burned) and decreasing intake (calories eaten). That's a lifestyle change. Try to find small ways to eat less and move more every day. You will be amazed at what happens over time. You cannot lose weight at the same pace you put it on. Most people could easily eat 2,000 calories or more in an hour. Yet as I said before, the average woman only burns 1,700 in a day. Have realistic expectations and always remember that every bite you choose to put in your mouth counts.

If your metabolism is average, your body will melt off close to a pound of fat per week if you follow the equation above. If you are too aggressive, burning an excess 700 to 1,000 calories a day above your intake (aka dieting), your metabolism may actually begin to slow down. The metabolic threshold is different for everyone. Some people's metabolisms are so sensitive (usually from excessive dieting) that they seem to slow down when they think about dieting. My point is that you will protect your metabolism and do a better job at developing lasting lifestyle habits if you don't go overboard. You are not on a diet; you are re-creating the way you live in your physical dimension. At the very least, you must eat the number of calories equal to your RMR (resting metabolic rate). For me that is about 1,400 calories.

To get a rough estimate of your RMR, go to www.bmi-calculator .net/bmr-calculator/ and plug in your personal stats. Remember that the answer will be based on an average metabolism. If you are extremely sedentary with little muscle mass, in actuality yours will be lower. If you are very active with lots of muscle, it will be higher than the estimation. No matter, use the number as the minimum number of calories you must eat to promote a healthy metabolism. Or for an even simpler estimate, multiply your weight times ten if you are fairly active, nine if you are only slightly active, and eight if you are extremely sedentary.

Now What?

If you've tracked with me thus far, I think you understand that you'll need to eat less and move more to burn excess fat. So how are you going to do that? I've already given you some very simple ideas, but I must say that the most accurate and effective method is calorie counting. I know that sounds like a diet, but it's not. It is simply getting educated on the caloric value of foods. It is also very enlightening to take a few average days and count how many calories you usually eat before you even attempt to cut back. People tell me all the time that they really don't eat very much. But when they sit down and list every single morsel they put in their mouth on a given day, they are really surprised at how fast the numbers add up.

Years ago I was teaching a lifestyle class on this subject and giving examples of how many calories are consumed eating common restaurant meals. From the back of the room I heard a gal cry out, "Oh my, that's why I'm so fat!" My point: we all need a reality check. We check the price on most items we purchase before we purchase them, but we rarely check the calories of the foods we eat. So, it makes sense to go to "calorie college" for six to eight weeks to become educated. It can make a huge impact. Some things taste really good, but when you find out the calorie count, you realize . . . they don't taste *that* good.

More Fat-Burning Facts

For those of you who are interested in the subject and want a little more knowledge, I've included a few more tips below. If not, that's okay. Just skip down to our next lifestyle area and pick up there.

My desire is to give you enough knowledge that you can apply it with wisdom and realize change. I caution those of you who are perfectionists to realize that you don't need to implement every suggestion. Find the two or three things that sound best to you and work on those first. Then, as you realize success, come back to this teaching and take action in more ways.

Eat and Burn All Day Long

Your body actually knows about how many calories it needs at specific times of day. If you don't fuel up right, it revolts with fatigue, cravings, and more efficient fat storage. But if you eat and burn all day long with frequent yet smaller meals and snacks, your body will respond with higher energy because it has sufficient, immediate fuel throughout the day. When we start seeing pounds sneak on our bodies, our first instinct is often to skip meals. Don't! As you learned earlier, cutting calories too dramatically can damage your metabolism. Even if you eat the same number of calories, you'll burn them off better if you spread them throughout the day. This is especially true for postmenopausal women, who find it easier to put weight on and harder to take it off. Most experts agree that women who eat larger meals instead of nutritious mini-meals may burn off sixty fewer calories a day. That means switching to mini-meals, spaced throughout the day, could save you from gaining six pounds a year.

Begin with Breakfast

Breakfast is the most important meal of the day. It stimulates your metabolism to get cooking early in the day and sets the stage for your energy level in the afternoon. In fact, studies show breakfast increases your metabolism by about 10 percent. That's huge!

What is a good breakfast? Always include a strong base of complex carbohydrates (full of fiber) that act as kindling to stoke your metabolic fire, balanced with moderate amounts of protein and smaller amounts of fat. Periodically stoking your fire all day long with this blend of foods will enhance your calorie-burning capability.

Overeating diverts large amounts of blood to your digestive tract and makes you feel sleepy and sluggish. That is why you get the "after-lunch blahs." So get lean and energized by eating more of your calories in the first twelve hours of your day when you burn them best! Try to avoid refined carbohydrates, sugars, and caffeine until after lunch when you have created a strong nutritional base of protein and fiber to stabilize your blood sugar. Begin to practice this discipline consistently, and it will help sugar cravings become a thing of the past.

As you renew your mind, it will get easier to deal with the mental and emotional issues that can influence you to overeat. I cover issues of emotional eating and eating disorders at length in *Scale Down*. Learning to delay gratification, tune into true hunger, and also identify your common eating triggers can be helpful in your quest for more effective fat management.

Activity and Exercise

The old cliché is true: if you don't use it, you'll lose it. You may eat quality foods and maintain a healthy weight, but if you lead a sedentary lifestyle, you are compromising your health and vitality. God gave us bones, muscles, joints, and ligaments because we were designed to move . . . a lot. Because of our advanced technology and expectation to accomplish so much in so little time, most of us need to purposely add activity into our lives. And, if we want to lose body fat, aerobic activity is especially important. You know that, I know that, but too often we put off exercise until tomorrow . . . and each tomorrow ends up being days or weeks away. As I sit writing this book (with a looming deadline of four weeks), I realize that I have not had a really good workout for three days. (I'm human too!) I am noticing a significant drop in my energy over the last day or so. I know what I teach is true: regular exercise creates a positive energy cycle. I think I'll take a break—to break a sweat in my little home gym downstairs. I'll be back shortly. You can take a spin around the block or do a few sit-ups right now too. Really, take a break and burn a few calories.

Okay . . . I'm back. Phew, I feel so much better.

You may not be an expert body builder or know all the latest facts about exercise physiology, but you do know how to move. So I've decided not to bore you with too much information. Instead, I'll remind you of a couple basics and encourage you to find creative ways to move as much as possible every day.

As I already mentioned, one of my favorite tools to motivate myself and others to increase activity is the Caltrac. In fact, mine told me that I just burned 420 activity calories during my 45-minute aerobic workout a little while ago. Whether you know how many calories you burn or not, you need to find little ways to remind yourself that all forms of movement add up and promote an active lifestyle.

In days past, people bent and stretched, lifted and loaded, working a variety of muscles in various ways all day long. They did not need to be told that the three important components of fitness include aerobic conditioning, muscle toning, and flexibility. Their lifestyles took care of all three. Since ours don't, we must be mindful to include them.

Small Steps Taken Consistently . . . Add Up!

To follow are some simple yet effective things you can incorporate into your life to address all three components of total fitness. Even on your busiest days, do something physical. We can all find ten or fifteen minutes here or there to burn a few calories or stretch or condition a muscle group.

Small Steps Toward Strengthened and Toned Muscles

Take a toning class or buy a good exercise video.

Consider a personal trainer for two or three sessions.

Buy a small variety of hand weights and learn some simple exercises you can do at home.

Learn some basic toning exercises that use only your body as weight that you can do anywhere.

Put abdominal strength at the top of your list. Learn and practice safe sit-ups at least three times a week. Strong abdominal muscles will support your lower back and improve your posture. When you stand tall with your stomach pulled in, you look ten pounds leaner!

Small Steps Toward Aerobic Endurance

Start with as little as fifteen minutes of low-intensity aerobic activity, three times a week. Gradually progress to a minimum of thirty minutes of moderately intense aerobic activity five or more times a week. Fat metabolism maximizes only during aerobic conditioning and reaches 50 percent of total calories being burned only after thirty minutes of aerobic activity.

Start each aerobic segment at a comfortable pace, allowing your cardiovascular system to adjust and your muscles to warm up fully.

Keep moving steadily for at least the first three minutes. Then, once the muscles are warm, take a few minutes to stretch key muscles you will be using during your workout. Then, resume your aerobic workout.

If you feel stiff or sore, slow your pace down and allow your heart rate and breathing to adjust to the activity.

Small Steps Toward a Flexible and Injury-Free Body

Incorporate a full body stretch into your fitness routine three or more times each week.

Always stretch after a two-to-five-minute, low-intensity aerobic warm-up when your muscles are warm and more stretchable and again after your cool down.

Stretch slowly without bouncing and hold each stretch for fifteen to thirty seconds, gradually releasing back to the starting position.

Pay special attention to hip, lower back, hamstring, and quadriceps muscle groups.

Tune in to your muscles. They will tell you what they need.

If you think you hate exercise, or constantly tell yourself that you don't have the time, then you will hate it and you won't make the time. Work at developing healthy attitudes that will move exercise from an attitude of "I have to, but I don't want to" to an attitude of "I need to and I want to." Here are some ways to do this.

Decide to make exercise a permanent part of your life.

Identify and work on any self-talk "speed bumps."

Set manageable and realistic goals.

Make an appointment with yourself daily . . . and keep it.

Select activities that you enjoy.

Incorporate strength, endurance, and flexibility into your routine.

Try cross training to maximize benefits and minimize injury.

If you can do only one thing—move aerobically.

Start out slowly.

Listen to your body.

Make it enjoyable so you will keep doing it day after day.

Realize that any exercise is better than no exercise at all.

Find and use fitness resources.

Use common sense and listen to your body as you strive to increase your activity and improve your fitness level. Many people make the mistake of working out first thing in the morning before eating anything. A light snack a few minutes beforehand will provide you with sufficient energy for the activity. Even if you don't like to eat in the morning, try to change that habit and take in 100–150 calories in a banana or nutrition bar. Your fat-burning efficiency is actually improved if your body is well fueled. Exercise does not have to be painful in order to be effective. You should notice an increased alertness and energy after a workout. If you don't, you may have worked too hard, too long, or without enough fuel.

As we close out our teaching on these three foundational lifestyle habits (nutrition, fat management, and exercise), I highly recommend that you read and repeat the following healthy statements below, in conjunction with putting some of these principles into practice. Thousands of my readers and clients have used my biblically grounded Healthy Self-Talk CDs to help them change their unhealthy thinking into God-honoring perspectives that move them toward healthier habits. Don't underestimate the power of truth to transform you from the inside out. Now, grab a pen and write down the ones that speak to you . . . and read them every day.

- I am finding creative ways to eat fewer calories every day.
- I am finding simple ways to burn more calories every day.
- I am learning to eat for maximum energy and health.
- I am making purposeful activity or exercise a regular habit.
- I am identifying and changing my unhealthy beliefs and attitudes.
- I am building a foundation of truth from God's Word.
- I am becoming transformed by the renewing of my mind.
- I am learning to see myself and my goals through God's eyes.

Rest and Regeneration

> Six days you shall labor and do all your work, but the seventh day is a Sabbath to the Lord your God. On it you shall not do any work.

> . . . For in six days the LORD made the heavens and the earth, the sea, and all that is in them, but he rested on the seventh day. Therefore the LORD blessed the Sabbath day and made it holy.
>
> Exodus 20:9–11

We have twenty-four hours in every day, and for some reason our bodies want to throw in the towel at about sixteen hours, demanding rest and sleep. Why in the world did God create us with bodies that fail us one-third of our day, only to repeat the same cycle the next day? I certainly can't answer that question; but I will ask him one day! I speculate that perhaps in part because it makes us acknowledge our own frailty and mortality. One thing I do know is that God in all his omnipotence did not personally need to take a break on the seventh day after all his work was done. He is the eternal, all-powerful Creator. So, we must conclude that he was modeling what he wanted us to practice. Not only do our bodies need rest, we need to break away from weekday busyness and completely worship the Lord with all of our hearts, souls, strength . . . and, oh yes . . . time.

We need rest to regenerate our bodies, souls, and spirits on a regular basis. God created us for daily rest, in addition to a weekly break from all of our toil. We need to relax our minds and bodies regularly or we pay a huge price in our mental and physical health. In my younger years I considered sleep a waste of time. I was juggling motherhood and career, believing the lie that I could be a superwoman, successful at every aspect if I just gave it "quality" time. I learned the hard way that quality alone does not make up for quantity . . . in our bodies, our relationships, or our intimacy with God.

Stress Kills

A healthy lifestyle must include adequate time for mental, emotional, and physical reprieve. This includes identifying and dealing with undue and persistent stress. If you are always feeling a sense of pressure day in and day out, stress that never abates for long, your body will be impacted in potentially harmful ways. Chronic stress must be evaluated and subjected to God's truth and dealt with in a biblical way. In his letter to the Philippians, Paul writes:

> Do not be anxious about anything, but in everything, by prayer and petition, with thanksgiving, present your requests to God. And the peace of God, which transcends all understanding, will guard your hearts and your minds in Christ Jesus.
>
> Philippians 4:6–7

How in the world can Paul expect us to be anxious for nothing? Doesn't he understand the kind of pressures and challenges we face day after day? I'm guessing he understood better than most people in light of the fact that he had been shipwrecked, beaten, and imprisoned multiple times. If anyone had credibility on the subject of anxiety or stress, it was Paul. And notice he doesn't even give us a short list of things we *should* be stressed about. He says be anxious for *nothing*! The good news is that he shows us exactly how we can accomplish that task. In the next sentence he gives us the biblical formula for finding peace despite the circumstances of life.

Notice that Paul uses the powerful word *but*. He means instead of being anxious, do something that matters. That something is in everything pray and petition with a heart of thanksgiving. Talk to God and share your heart. Rather than giving in to anxiety and stress, take hold of the promise. And the peace of God, which transcends all understanding, will guard your heart and your mind in Christ Jesus. Your part is to identify your stressful thoughts and stop yourself from stewing and worrying. Always look up and set your mind on God. Thank him for who he is and what he has done, then receive the peace that comes only when you walk in his Spirit. This is how we move from the flesh to abiding in Christ, which is one and the same as walking in the Spirit. We can practice this principle in every area of our lives. It's a shift of perspective from flesh to spirit. When we by our own free will choose to do this, his peace is the supernatural gift we receive.

Overscheduled . . . Overtired

One of the reasons we are so stressed and never feel relaxed and regenerated is because we overschedule our lives. Too many of us rarely have a day without commitments. We run from activity to activity until we collapse in bed for a night of restless sleep. God did not design us to be constantly on the go. We need moments of quiet and peace each day. If you study Christ's life, you read over and over how he got away to be alone with God. And though he told his disciples to pick up their crosses and follow him (to give up their total lives to him alone), he recognized their need for rest. Here are his words to the men he so loved:

> And He said to them, "Come away by yourselves to a secluded place and rest a while." (For there were many people coming and going, and they did not even have time to eat.)
>
> Mark 6:31 NASB

For all of us who carry the worry and burdens of life like heavy sacks of sand on our shoulders, Jesus calls us to physical, mental, emotional, and spiritual rest.

> Come to Me, all you who labor and are heavy laden, and I will give you rest. Take my yoke upon you and learn from Me, for I am gentle and lowly in heart, and you will find rest for your souls.
>
> Matthew 11:28–29 NASB

Sleep

Sleep is the time when you get both physical and psychological rest. During deep sleep, your body accomplishes its most important cellular renewal. Even modest amounts of sleep deprivation can diminish your immune system and ability to cope with the daily challenges of life. If you want to look younger, feel better, and live longer—get enough sleep! How much is enough? Experts suggest that most people need close to eight hours of sleep every night.

I have found that chronic fatigue is one of the biggest factors influencing lack of self-control. We lose our resolve and give in to our weaknesses when we are exhausted. For those who struggle with overeating, a fatigued body seems to say, "If you're not going to give me enough quality rest to reenergize, I'm just going to beg for sugar and calories all day long to make up for it!" My suggestion: make sleep a priority. Try getting eight hours of sleep a night for a full month and see the impact it makes in your lifestyle.

Like eating well and being physically active, getting a good night's sleep is vital to your well-being.

Here are a few tips to help you get a good night's sleep:

Get adequate exposure to sunlight. Your body needs to experience daylight to regulate normal sleep patterns. Try to spend at least thirty minutes each day outside in natural light.

Stick to a regular sleep schedule. Try to go to bed and wake up at the same time each day; even weekends if at all possible.

Avoid large meals and beverages late at night. A large meal requires much digestive activity, not to mention causes indigestion, which can interfere with sleep. Drinking too many fluids at night can cause you to awaken frequently to urinate and then perhaps have difficulty falling back to sleep.

Stay away from stimulants like caffeine. The stimulating effects of caffeine in coffee, colas, teas, and chocolate take up to six hours to wear off completely.

Avoid alcoholic drinks before bed. A little wine may help you get to sleep but will not allow you to fall into the deep stages of sleep. Many people tend to wake up in the middle of the night once the sedating effects have worn off.

Relax before bed. You need to tell your mind and body that you are approaching bedtime. Engage in a relaxing activity, such as reading or listening to music, and avoid books or television programs that elicit strong emotions.

Take a hot bath before bed. Baths are very relaxing, and the drop in body temperature after the bath can help you fall asleep more readily. Try a little candlelight during your bath for an even better sleep-inducing effect.

Create a positive sleep environment. A quiet, dark room and comfortable bed are essentials for a good night's sleep. Avoid watching TV or working on a computer thirty to sixty minutes before you want to go to sleep. Keeping the temperature in your bedroom on the cool side enhances sleep.

Don't lie in bed awake. When you can't get to sleep or back to sleep within twenty minutes, get up and do some relaxing activity until you feel sleepy. Reading something enjoyable but nontaxing can be helpful. Anxiety about falling asleep can make it more difficult to do it. Go back to bed when you feel groggy.

Seek medical help if you consistently find yourself feeling tired during the day despite spending enough time in bed at night, as you may have a sleep disorder.

Destructive Habits and Attitudes

While poor nutrition, overeating, lack of sleep, and an overbusy lifestyle can negatively impact your life on many levels, some habits and addictions can seem to almost possess you. Severe eating disorders, smoking, excessive drinking, too much shopping or gambling, drug addiction, or pornography have destroyed the lives of too many people, including too many Christians.

I am not an expert on any of these destructive habits, though I have certainly been in the pit of despair because of my own. However, I am well grounded in the truth of Scripture and God's ability to renew even the most desperate heart and mind. My main purpose in addressing issues such as these is to make sure that those of you who struggle do not continue to hide them in a closet and live in shame any longer.

One of the things that gave me great comfort in the days that I was emerging from my eating disorder and other destructive habits was studying the life of King David. As I read many of his psalms, I could identify as he poured out his heart to God. It says in Scripture that David was a man after God's own heart (Acts 13:22). God chose him to be king. Yet if you've read of his life, you know that he sinned against God grievously by taking Bathsheba (another man's wife), getting her pregnant, and then having her husband killed to cover his sin. You can't get much more shameful than that. As king, David could do as he pleased because he had incredible power. But when his good friend Nathan had the courage to confront him, David was humbled and convicted of his sin. You can almost hear his heart breaking as he calls out to God in Psalm 51:1–12:

> Have mercy on me, O God,
> according to your unfailing love;
> according to your great compassion
> blot out my transgressions.
> Wash away all my iniquity
> and cleanse me from my sin.
> For I know my transgressions,
> and my sin is always before me.
> Against you, you only, have I sinned
> and done what is evil in your sight;
> so that you are proved right when you speak
> and justified when you judge.
> Surely I was sinful at birth,
> sinful from the time my mother conceived me.
> Surely you desire truth in the inner parts;
> you teach me wisdom in the inmost place.
> Cleanse me with hyssop, and I will be clean;
> wash me, and I will be whiter than snow.

> Let me hear joy and gladness;
> let the bones you have crushed rejoice.
> Hide your face from my sins
> and blot out all my iniquity.
> Create in me a pure heart, O God,
> and renew a steadfast spirit within me.
> Do not cast me from your presence
> or take your Holy Spirit from me.
> Restore to me the joy of your salvation
> and grant me a willing spirit, to sustain me.

It is extremely important to note that in the days when David prayed this prayer, the Holy Spirit did not reside within believers. He would come and go often depending on the condition of a person's heart. Today, as New Testament believers, we can greatly grieve the Holy Spirit, but he never leaves us. And, like David, we must call out to God from our pain—broken and humbled—and he will restore our joy and grant us a willing spirit. That is the only thing that can fully sustain us.

Just praying this prayer over and over does not mean that you will necessarily be healed immediately from your habit or addiction. But it does mean that God will answer your prayers and bring resources and people around you to walk you through the long and often painful path to recovery.

One of my dearest friends in the entire world, Sylvia Lange, knows what it is like to be lost in the pit of despair. I think her story, told in her own words, will encourage you.[4]

Sylvia's Story

From as far back as I can remember, I never felt that I measured up to anyone's expectations, least of all mine. I believed that the "real me" wasn't good enough, so I would make up different personas to appeal to each person or situation I encountered in a feeble attempt to simply feel normal. As a result, a hole began to grow in the center of my soul at a very young age. I learned how to live a total lie, lying to just about everyone. As I got older, I became a downright expert in this charade in my desperate attempt to feel accepted and loved.

Over time, the hole grew larger and larger as I totally lost sight of who I really was in the empty, phony life I had chosen. As the years dragged on, I tried everything I could to fill up that hole because I couldn't stand myself as I was. I tried therapy, spending hundreds of hours and thousands of dollars only to sit in a therapist's office and lie about what was really happening in my life.

Another feeble attempt to feel normal was through dating seemingly every available man I met in my search for love. With every one of those relationships, I would give pieces of myself away, further enlarging the hole.

I also tried church. I remember fully accepting who Christ was in my mind, but feeling nothing in my spirit. I've often heard that the farthest distance in the world is between our heads and our hearts. I would go to church on Sunday and have a compelling experience in the church pew, only to return home to an unchanged life. Often, I would spend the rest of the day in my bed, unable to get up until I had to go to work the next morning. I was totally crippled by my depression.

In my late twenties, I discovered in social situations that a glass of wine would take the edge off, calm me down. So I'd have a second, and by the end of it, I felt as "normal" as I perceived everyone around me to be. But by the third or the fourth glass, I would begin to make a fool of myself, and because I couldn't stand for anyone to think badly of me, I took that growing problem underground. It became the latest secret I kept from all my good church friends. Day after day, I would come home from a fourteen-hour day, drink a bottle of something, and pass out on my couch. I would pull myself together the next morning and do it all over again. I kept this cycle up for years. I believe I was a full-blown alcoholic by the time

I was thirty years old. I could barely say the word, I was so ashamed! But I managed to hold it all together in public, especially in front of my church friends, as I pretended to be the epitome of a good, religious person.

Shame had become my constant companion in every area of my life as I compromised myself in dating relationships, cut corners at work, and lied to family and friends. Then one night I came to the end of the asphalt. I felt as low as I could ever remember. I came home from work that night, dropped my keys on the floor, and went straight to bed, too drained to even go into the kitchen and pour a glass of comfort as I did every other night. As I lay there in the darkness, it suddenly hit me—this is what it feels like to want to die.

Nothing I had tried had worked. Not therapy, not men, not church, not even the drinking—nothing. The thought must've scared me, because I remember getting out of my bed, and before I knew it, I was at the door of a neighbor whom I really didn't know but who appeared to be living an authentic life. On this particular night, I awoke Margaret and her husband late in the night. They were surprised to see me, but as I blurted out, "I need to talk," they warmly invited me in. Throughout the night, I poured out my soul and told them things I'd never told a pastor, a friend, my mother, absolutely no one. And all the judgment I expected from good people like that never came. They simply loved on me as one secret after another came pouring out. The relief that began to wash over me was extraordinary. It was like the weight of the world was lifted off my shoulders with every hideous confession. Today I understand what happened that night. James 5:16 encourages us to confess our stuff to each other—tell the truth to another human being; not for forgiveness but for healing. I believe my healing began that night as I told the truth for the very first time.

In the early hours of the morning when I was all "talked out," Margaret turned to me and said something that I will never forget. She said, "Sylvia, do you have any idea how much Jesus loves you?"

I swear to you, if she had asked me that one day earlier, I am certain I would've dismissed it as one of the trite things I thought church people were supposed to say. But this time, it hit me: she was talking about the God of the universe, and that he loved . . . me. The power of that hit me like a ton of bricks, and suddenly I got it. I was loved, just as I was, by a holy God.

That night was the last time I felt the need to take a drink to fill the hole in my gut, and although life hasn't been perfect since then (how could it be . . . *I'm* still here), it is honest, and I feel peace. I truly do. Through the help of a twelve-step recovery program, the support of friends and family, the power of God's Word through the Scriptures, and the mind-blowing love of God himself, my life today is very different. I have learned that without God at the center of my life, it is all an exercise in futility. I need his Spirit's power and the help and accountability of mature people who have walked this road ahead of me. Today, my life is fueled by gratitude as I live under the pure grace of God. Over the last nine years, I have learned that by rigorously following these twelve steps that I learned as part of a Christian Twelve-Step Program, I can actually live the "abundant life" Jesus said in John 10:10 that he came to offer.

Step 1 is about recognizing our brokenness. We admitted that we were powerless over the effects of our separation from God—that our lives had become unmanageable. "I know that nothing good lives in me, that is, in my sinful nature. For I have the desire to do what is good, but I cannot carry it out" (Rom. 7:18).

Step 2 is about the birth of faith in us. Came to believe that a power greater than ourselves can restore us to sanity. "For it is God who works in you to will and to act according to his good purpose" (Phil. 2:13).

Step 3 involves a decision to let God be in charge of our lives. Made a decision to turn our will and our lives over to the care of God as we understood him. "Therefore, I urge you, brothers, in view of God's mercy, to offer your bodies as living sacrifices, holy and pleasing to God—this is your spiritual act of worship" (Rom. 12:1).

Step 4 involves self-examination. Made a searching and fearless moral inventory of ourselves. "Let us examine our ways and test them, and let us return to the LORD" (Lam. 3:40).

Step 5 is the discipline of confession. Admitted to God, to ourselves, and to another human being the exact nature of our wrongs. "Therefore confess your sins to each other and pray for each other so that you may be healed" (James 5:16).

Step 6 is an inner transformation sometimes called repentance. Were entirely ready to have God remove all these defects of character. "Humble yourselves before the Lord, and he will lift you up" (James 4:10).

Step 7 involves the transformation or purification of our character. Humbly asked God to remove our shortcomings. "If we confess our sins, he is faithful and just and will forgive us our sins and purify us from all unrighteousness" (1 John 1:9).

Step 8 involves examining our relationships and preparing ourselves to make amends. Made a list of all persons we had harmed and became willing to make amends to them all. "Do to others as you would have them do to you" (Luke 6:31).

Step 9 is the discipline of making amends. Made direct amends to such people wherever possible, except when to do so would injure them or others. "Therefore, if you are offering your gift at the altar and there remember that your brother has something against you, leave your gift there in front of the altar. First go and be reconciled to your brother; then come and offer your gift" (Matt. 5:23–24).

Step 10 is about maintaining progress in recovery. Continued to take personal inventory, and when we were wrong, promptly admitted it. "So, if you think you are standing firm, be careful that you don't fall!" (1 Cor. 10:12).

Step 11 involves the spiritual disciplines of prayer and meditation. Sought through prayer and meditation to improve our conscious contact with God as we understand him, praying only for the knowledge of his will for us and the power to carry that out. "Let the word of Christ dwell in you richly" (Col. 3:16).

Step 12 is about ministry. Having had a spiritual awakening as the result of these steps, tried to carry this message to others, and to practice these principles in all our affairs. "Brothers, if someone is caught in a sin, you who are spiritual should restore him gently. But watch yourself, or you also may be tempted" (Gal. 6:1).[5]

We all need help in life. Yet, our pride gets in the way. Again we can learn from David, who called out to God multiple times in his human frailty and failure. Don't keep silent any longer. Confess your sin to a trustworthy, mature Christian or counselor. Call out to God and begin the process of restoration today.

> When I kept silent,
> my bones wasted away
> through my groaning all day long.
> For day and night
> your hand was heavy upon me;
> my strength was sapped
> as in the heat of summer.
> Then I acknowledged my sin to you
> and did not cover up my iniquity.
> I said, "I will confess
> my transgressions to the Lord"—
> and you forgave
> the guilt of my sin.
>
> Psalm 32:3–5

a forty-day strategy toward permanent change

> God's training is for now, not later. His purpose is for this very minute, not for sometime in the future. We have nothing to do with what will follow our obedience, and we are wrong to concern ourselves with it. What people call preparation, God sees as the goal itself.[1]
>
> Oswald Chambers

God's purpose is for this very minute, for the sixty minutes in every hour, the twenty-four hours in every day. If we are obedient by doing "the right things for the right reasons," then we must trust him with the results. His principles always prevail. I love that this famous (now deceased) author reminds us that God sees the process we live right now as the goal, an end in itself. How we choose minute to minute matters to him. We cannot do anything about yesterday. And tomorrow is not yet here. This very day, we must choose how we will think and act. If we think about God and act upon his proven plan for healthy living, the process and our obedience will surely produce good fruit.

In this chapter, I will explain the process I've designed for the daily portion of this book as well as the four personal evaluations at the end of this chapter. It is important to take those before you begin your forty-day journey. Then, beginning tomorrow (or when you finish the evaluations), you can start with day 1.

Each Day Has Three Important Components

Nourish your spirit
Nourish your soul
Nourish your body

It is ideal if you can spend about ten minutes early in the day reading and reflecting on the nourish your spirit and soul section and then five to ten minutes at the end of your day logging and planning for tomorrow. It is my hope that you will continue for forty consecutive days without any breaks. But, if you miss a day, quickly pick up where you left off.

Nourish Your Spirit

Each day includes a devotion based on the key Scripture of the day. It is concluded with a prayer. The prayer is only an example. If it speaks words that resonate with your heart, by all means read it as a prayer to God. If not, pray as you are led.

Nourish Your Soul

This section follows the devotion and gives you an opportunity to process some of your own thoughts immediately. Use it as a time of reflection to grow in the area of renewing your mind. I have included a completed example below (to a nonexistent devotion) to help illustrate.

FROM THE DEVOTION ABOVE I HAVE IDENTIFIED . . .

The lie I believe:

I believe I am a failure and that God is ashamed of me.

The truth I now receive:

God loves me and wants to give me freedom in Christ. He is on my side. I can go to Him despite my behavior as His love is secure.

☒ ☒ ☒ I practiced healthy self-talk today (1 to 3 times).

My key personal statement is:

God loves me just as I am and wants me to run to Him in my weakness. When I feel ashamed, I call on His name and He is there.

☒ ☒ ☒ I have repeated that message at least 3 times today.

☒ I have written my personal statement above on an index card or in my new self-talk notebook that I can continue to read if I need renewal in this area.

Keep It Simple

Don't let the process of putting down your thoughts become a burden. If after a moment of thinking about it, you have nothing to say, then leave it blank. Some days will speak to you more than others. When you write a key personal statement, phrase it in a way that will speak power and truth into your mind. Don't write "I am not a failure," but rather "Through God's power I am victorious in all things." If you write a statement that really resonates with you, put it on an index card or a small self-talk notebook that you can easily refer to again and again. Obviously you will check the boxes indicating if you practiced healthy self-talk or repeated your personal statements at the end of the day. If you are not accustomed to journaling or logging, at least give it a try, as it can be a very effective tool.

Healthy Self-Talk Is Essential

The daily exercise above may help you write your own healthy self-talk statements. The daily devotional Scriptures may help you identify key Scripture that speak to you in your area of struggle or pain. Over time you will collect both personal statements and Scripture that can become very important for your journey. Keep collecting and reading these. At a point, you can thin down your collection to those that are most important to you. At the end of the forty days, choose the top five to ten and find time each and every day to read and speak them aloud. As I mentioned in chapter 2, you can also make your own CD or use mine, as that is a very time-efficient way to fill your mind with truth.

Nourish Your Body

Each day, I will provide you with a short segment that addresses healthy living and is intended to inspire or educate you in practical ways. It is followed by a logging section that you should complete at the end of each day so you can record your lifestyle habits for that day. It is one way of making you accountable to yourself and watching your progress day to day. Don't become a slave to the process. If there is a particular area that you simply don't need to address, then don't. Make the process work for you. Decide what is important and then commit to that. I have included a completed example below. At the very end, there is a place to record your thoughts for the day.

DAILY JOURNAL & LOG

My unhealthy habit(s) is diminishing and my new habits are increasing in the following ways:

Just by taking action, I feel like I am finally doing something healthy about my habit of emotional eating. Knowing that I have a forty-day journey to guide me and keep me focused on all I've learned gives me hope as I start implementing what I have learned.

Nutrition & Fat Management

I ate for maximum energy and health today in the following ways:

☒ By drinking 4 to 6 ounces of water most waking hours

☒ By eating protein and/or fiber at breakfast.

☒ By eating 3 to 4 vegetables. This is hard for me

☒ By eating 2 to 3 fruits, whole grains or nuts. Ate only 1 serving

☒ By eating 5 to 6 snacks or small meals. Ate 4 small meals

☒ By eating less from bags and boxes. Another hard thing

☒ By eating only when I was hungry. Did great today!

☒ By eating 20 to 50 percent less food than usual in the last four hours of the day. This works well

☒ By eating no more than 10 percent "empty" calories. Not sure, ate a cookie

Rest and Regeneration

Last night I slept 6 hours. The quality of my sleep was: OK

To ensure I get quality rest tonight I will turn off the TV earlier.

Today I managed my stress by saying no to another committee

Tomorrow I will unwind and relax by leaving work on time and going for a walk

☒ I practiced deep breathing today for relaxation and health.

Fitness

☒ Today I did my minimum ten minutes of exercise.

I exceeded the minimum by 20 minutes—YEAH!!!

Tomorrow I will improve or maintain my fitness by buying and using light weights.

Thoughts for Today

It seems like this process is easy enough to stick with until my mind catches up with my actions. I need to let go of perfection and feeling pressure to check off everything on the logging list every day.

Personal Evaluations

The personal evaluations that follow are simply tools to help you identify your weak spots in each lifestyle category before you begin your forty-day journey. Rate yourself as honestly as you can. No one else needs to see this. Notice that the statements in the personal evaluations are all phrased in a positive bent and may be helpful to you in developing your own personal statements, which we'll discuss more after you've completed each evaluation.

Mental and Spiritual Habits Evaluation

Based on the last three months, please rate yourself (0—almost never; 1—sometimes; 2—often; 3—always).

___ I see myself as a fully accepted and loved child of God.
___ My choices and actions are mostly based on my desire to honor God.
___ I am thankful for the body and mind God has given me.
___ I usually try to honor God with my lifestyle habits.
___ I see my body as a gift from God and take responsibility for my health.
___ My attitude is this: I am not my behavior. I am complete in Christ.
___ I surrender my weaknesses to God and rely on his strength for the moment.
___ My personal goals are realistic and honor God.
___ I take realistic steps toward my goals each day.
___ I know that with God's help, I can overcome my habits and have a healthy mind and body.
___ I am aware of the lies I believe about my body, health, and habits and now tell myself the truth.
___ I recognize when my thinking is unhealthy and take positive action to change it.
___ I renew my mind with God's truth each day.
___ I am a work in progress and try to give myself grace as I pursue lasting change.
___ Each day, I choose to submit my body, mind, and spirit to God.

___ I pray daily for God's power to walk in the Spirit and not fulfill the desires of my flesh.

___ **Add the total of all scores.**

Scoring

48–40 Excellent! You have a godly perspective.

39–31 Good. Your perspective is usually healthy.

30–22 Fair. It's time to get a new focus . . . the truth!

< 22 Alert! Alert! Change your thinking immediately!

Nutritional Habits Evaluation

Based on the last three months, please rate yourself (0—almost never; 1—sometimes; 2—often; 3—always).

___ I think about what I eat and how it impacts my health.

___ I have high energy to do all the things I want and need to do.

___ I read labels and choose many foods based on that information.

___ I eat two to three servings of fruit each day.

___ I eat three to four servings of vegetables each day.

___ I choose whole-grain products over more processed foods.

___ I know how much fiber I'm eating daily.

___ I drink an average of four to eight ounces of water each hour I am awake.

___ I eat a healthy breakfast with fiber in it every day.

___ I eat a good source of protein at breakfast.

___ I choose and eat lean protein with my lunch.

___ I limit my empty calories to less than 10 to 15 percent of my total diet.

___ I limit caffeine and other stimulants such as over-the-counter diet aids.

___ I take a multivitamin supplement daily.

___ I take an antioxidant supplement daily.
___ I eat healthy omega-3 fats daily and limit saturated fats.
___ **Add the total of all scores.**

Scoring

48–40 Excellent! Your body loves you!
39–31 Good. You're on the right track.
30–22 Fair. It's time to try a little more high-octane fuel.
< 22 Poor. Your body is crying "Help!"

Fat Management Habits Evaluation

Based on the past three months, please rate yourself (0—almost never; 1—sometimes; 2—often; 3—always).

___ I feel in control of my food choices.
___ I measure my size by how I look and feel, not the scale.
___ I eat only when I'm hungry.
___ I stop eating when I'm full.
___ I understand why calories count.
___ I eat four to five small meals or snacks per day.
___ I limit my junk food, fast food, and desserts to less than 15 percent of my diet.
___ I am happy with my body weight.
___ I am happy with my size and shape.
___ I can enjoy "fun food" in moderation without feeling guilty.
___ I think about food only when I'm hungry.
___ I can see myself eating and living in control.
___ I walk or get purposeful exercise at least four times per week.
___ I am very aware of my choices and how they affect my body.
___ I say no to the latest diets or supplements promising quick results.

___ I know if I'm going to be lean, I have to take daily action.
___ **Add the total of all scores.**

Scoring

48–40	Excellent! You've got a lean lifestyle.
39–31	Good. You're doing most things right!
30–22	Fair. It's time to take action.
< 22	Poor. Start with one step at a time.

Activity and Exercise Habits Evaluation

Based on the last three months, please rate yourself (0—almost never; 1—sometimes; 2—often; 3—always).

___ I crave activity and find ways to move throughout my day.
___ I enjoy exercise and how it makes my body feel.
___ I have high energy to do all the things I want and need to do.
___ I make exercise and activity a priority in my life.
___ I understand the need for aerobic, strength, and flexibility training.
___ I engage in aerobic activity four or more times per week.
___ I take the stairs or park far away whenever I can.
___ I monitor my heart rate and know I am exercising safely.
___ I am injury free and able to engage in most activities.
___ Being healthy and fit is important to me.
___ I listen to my body and know what it needs.
___ I wear appropriate and quality shoes for exercise.
___ I can walk at a fast pace and still carry on a conversation.
___ I work out my major muscle groups two to three times each week.
___ I can easily touch my toes without bending my knees.
___ I maintain strong abdominal muscles.
___ **Add the total of all scores.**

Scoring

48–40 Excellent! You're a fit machine!

39–31 Good. Stay consistent.

30–22 Fair. Use it or lose it!

< 22 Poor. Take one small step and start moving!

Now that you have completed all your evaluations, go back and circle with a red or blue pen all the "0" and "1" responses in each category. Now, write the statement correlating to that answer on an index card or in your "self-talk" notebook. Because these statements are all made in the affirmative, you can use them to "talk to yourself" in a more constructive way. At first you will feel as if you are telling yourself a lie. That is because you've been thinking and doing the opposite for far too long. Each day you can choose your focus. Don't choose to focus on your failures but rather on your potential for success.

You may have noticed that I did not include a "destructive habits" evaluation. You already know what those are. For those of you who are dealing with something in this category, please take a bold step and write your habit below. Perhaps you are open about such a habit and have already begun to ask family and friends for prayer and are seeking mature godly counsel. If you have not taken any steps and have been perhaps hiding your sin in secret, please not only write it below but also tell someone you can trust in the next few days. Then, write their name and the date next to your entry. There is something very powerful about facing off your sin.

For the rest of you, I encourage you to write the habit(s) you desire to change below before you begin the forty-day journey. Include any thoughts you may have as you surrender your body, soul, and spirit to the Lord.

____

____

____

____

____

____

Now that you have honestly evaluated yourself and written down your area of struggle, it is time to begin your daily journey. It will be forty days that will build a solid foundation for you to surrender your habits to God and allow him to begin the process of renewing your mind and transforming your life.

PART 2

the daily walk

a forty-day journey to nourish your spirit and nourish your body

day 1

Nourish Your Spirit—Drop the Stone

> "Woman, where are they? Has no one condemned you?" "No one, sir," she said. "Then neither do I condemn you," Jesus declared. "Go now and leave your life of sin."
>
> John 8:10–11

Here I go again . . . giving in to all my cravings and eating like there is no tomorrow. What is wrong with me? I remember the knot in my gut as I made comments like this one almost every day when I was struggling with emotional eating and bulimia. And I hear this kind of statement from people all over the country as I speak and share my story. They are frustrated and discouraged because they keep falling back into old patterns. Often they are stuck because they've become incredibly skilled at self-condemnation.

If you feel defeated and condemned to a life of bondage, who do you think is condemning you? I can assure you that your sense of shame is not of the Lord. He wants you to fully experience the power and freedom of your identity in him alone. In John 8, we read about a woman who was caught in the act of adultery. Yet, she was not condemned by Jesus. He showed her that even her accusers—the self-righteous Pharisees who wanted to stone her—were not without sin. In fact, they were not righteous enough to even cast the first stone.

This "woman of shame" lay at the feet of Jesus, exposed in all her sin. I can only imagine what she was waiting for him to do or say as the religious hypocrites slithered away, leaving her alone and face-to-face with the Lord. Did he remind her of all her failures? Did he condemn her for her sin? Did he wag his finger in contempt? No, he simply said, "Go and sin no more."

I have to believe that something supernatural happened in the heart of that woman in that moment. According to Jewish law, she should have been stoned to death. And now she was walking away free. But she was not just free from death, she was free from the bondage of her old life. While she could have gone back to her adulterous ways, I have to believe she was too profoundly transformed to live in that kind of bondage any longer. Jesus had not just spared her life, he had set her free from the lies she believed. He showed her that she was not alone in sin. He showed her the power of his profound grace. When she received him, her sin was washed away. She was no longer defined by her behavior but rather reborn in newness of life.

Don't get me wrong. I'm not saying that the Lord approved of her lifestyle. What I am saying is that condemnation and shame often send us into hiding and keep us in bondage.

When the Holy Spirit deals with us, it is with a conviction that brings repentance and a change in behavior that is rooted in right thinking and a pure heart. What does it take for each of us to move from self-condemnation to conviction and then lasting change that is rooted in truth? It takes faith and trust. We must believe that we are not "condemned" by God for our "bad" behavior. And we must stop condemning ourselves. We must trust that his truth alone will truly set us free. If we simply struggle by our own willpower and self-discipline to be "good," we will ultimately fail. But, if our motives are to surrender to him and to let him transform us into his image, we will discover incredible peace, power, and life-changing freedom.

If you are feeling defeated this very day by your failures, I am guessing that you are throwing stones at yourself. And, you probably have a great supporter (though truly an enemy) cheering you along. Put down the stones and listen to Jesus. Listen to him tell you how much he loves you (despite your behavior). He alone can give you the power to walk away from anything that holds you in bondage. Let go. Drop the stone. Grab his hand.

Prayer

Dear Lord, it is so true. I am hard on myself some days. I give in to a small temptation, and the next thing I know, I am out of control. The shame of feeling like a failure further diminishes my ability to dig myself out of my emotional rut and resume healthier ways. Please help me to "put down the stones." Help me to truly believe Romans 8:1, which says, "Therefore, there is now no condemnation for those who are in Christ Jesus." Help me to walk this day with you as my strength and my encourager. Amen.

FROM THE DEVOTION ABOVE I HAVE IDENTIFIED . . .

The lie I believe:

The truth I now receive:

☐ ☐ ☐ I practiced healthy self-talk today (one to three times).

My key personal statement is:

☐ ☐ ☐ I have repeated that message at least three times today.

☐ I have written my personal statement above on an index card or in a journal that I can continue to read if I need renewal in this area.

Nourish Your Body—Breathe

If you were stranded on a deserted island, you could potentially survive for months without food (depending on your fat reserves) but only two to three days without water. However, no matter where you are, the thing you need most to survive is air. From our first breath until our last, our bodies require a constant supply of oxygen. Yet, most of us are not breathing properly and thus diminishing our health in significant ways. Just because you are not turning blue does not mean your body is fully oxygenated. As children we laugh, run, and play in ways that encourage us to breathe deeply. In contrast, most adults breathe mostly from the upper chest, and many do not challenge their lungs frequently or sufficiently to maximize the life-enhancing benefits of deep breathing.

Improving your breathing techniques and increasing your respiratory capacity can decrease your blood pressure, heart rate, and level of stress in measurable ways. It can also improve your sleep, decrease your muscle tension, and increase your concentration.

On an even deeper level, deep breathing actually increases your immunity and helps remove toxins from your body by stimulating your lymphatic system to do its job more efficiently. Your circulatory system delivers nutrients and oxygen to your cells, and your lymphatic system carries those toxins away. But unlike your arteries, vessels, and capillaries that receive their nutrition from the pumping action of your heart, the lymphatic system is propelled by deep breathing and muscular contractions. It is essential to health as it is a key "sewage removal" system on the cellular level. Without it, we would die of toxicity within a day. Additionally, a healthy system is instrumental in maintaining a healthy immune system, which can destroy foreign cells such as cancer.

You can imagine how inefficient the lymphatic system must be for people who get little or no exercise and who rarely stimulate their body to breathe deeply from the diaphragm. By doing both on a daily basis, you can enhance your health tremendously. If you spend much of your day sitting, get up at least once an hour and move about for at least two to three minutes. Try to begin doing purposeful exercise that gets your heart beating faster and your respirations deeper at least four times a week.

Another very simple technique is to practice deep breathing for one to two minutes, three times per day. It is so simple you can do it while you are driving, watching television, or doing almost anything. When you first inhale, let your belly expand as you take about two seconds to completely fill your lungs. Then hold that air in for about four to five seconds, and lastly breathe out slowly until your lungs are empty for about four seconds. Repeat this exercise a total of ten times. This is such a simple habit that costs you nothing but can pay you in great health dividends. Breathe!

DAILY JOURNAL & LOG

My unhealthy habit(s) is diminishing and my new habits are increasing in the following ways:

Nutrition and Fat Management

I ate for maximum energy and health today in the following ways:

- ☐ By drinking 4 to 6 ounces of water most waking hours.
- ☐ By eating protein and/or fiber at breakfast.
- ☐ By eating 3 to 4 vegetables.
- ☐ By eating 2 to 3 servings of fruits, whole grains, or nuts.

☐ By eating 5 to 6 snacks or small meals.

☐ By eating less from bags and boxes.

☐ By eating only when I was hungry.

☐ By eating 20 to 50 percent less food than usual in the last 4 hours of the day.

☐ By eating no more than 10 percent "empty" calories.

Rest and Regeneration

Last night I slept ____________ hours.

The quality of my sleep was: ________________

Tonight I will ______________________________ to ensure I get quality rest.

Today I managed my stress by:

Tomorrow I will unwind and relax by:

☐ I practiced deep breathing today for relaxation and health.

Fitness

☐ Today I did my minimum 10 minutes of exercise.

I exceeded the minimum by ____________________

Tomorrow I will improve or maintain my fitness by:

Thoughts for Today

day 2

Nourish Your Spirit—Tempted

> Because he himself suffered when he was tempted, he is able to help those who are being tempted.
>
> Hebrews 2:18

The tall, attractive man in his late thirties stood before his Sunday school class and began to speak. There was bit of a catch in his voice as if he was having difficulty getting the words to come out. He said, "We get our cars tuned up. But how often do we get our marriages tuned up? I never gave much thought to that. I figured my marriage was fine. Then before I realized how little attention I'd given it, how out of tune it was, I found myself in an affair with another woman. Men, we are vulnerable. We need to strengthen our marriages and our relationship to Christ. Don't think you are immune. I thought I was. Fortunately that was a year ago. My wife has forgiven me, and I have rededicated my life to the Lord. So, how are you doing?"

When Christians who have fallen are willing to repent and surrender themselves to the Lord, he does amazing things in restoring their brokenness. And these restored people can become a great source of help to others. It is good to learn from the failings of others and know that God stands ready to bring us out of the pit of sin and despair. But we have an even better source of strength, one who was tempted but never sinned—Jesus.

In the desert, Satan taunted Jesus, telling him to turn the stones to bread. Jesus was very hungry for he had not eaten for forty days and he had the power to do as Satan asked. Instead he responded by saying, "It is written: 'Man does not live on bread alone, but on every word that comes from the mouth of God'" (Matt. 4:4). Satan made three attempts to throw Jesus off course, and all three times Jesus counteracted with Scripture—Scripture he had hidden in his heart.

When we are tempted, Jesus wants to help us. Like him, we need to turn to Scripture in our time of weakness. We can also turn to prayer. In the Garden of Gethsemane, Jesus knew he was going to die very soon and carry the sin of all humanity to the grave. He said to his disciples: "My soul is overwhelmed with sorrow to the point of death" (Mark 14:34). Then as he was praying he cried out to God, "*Abba*, Father, everything is possible for you. Take this cup from me. Yet not what I will, but what you will" (Mark 14:36).

Jesus could have surrendered to his own flesh and walked away. Instead, he surrendered to God.

We too must surrender our weakness and temptation to God, praying like Jesus, "Yet not my will, but yours be done." It is in humility and surrender that the power of the risen Christ can strengthen us from all temptations. When we choose to seek God and his power, he will meet us at our point of need.

Prayer

> Oh God, how I need your power and strength in times of temptation. I pray that the first thing that will come to my mind in those times will be your Word, and a desire to call out to you in prayer. Please help me make that my first response to each and every temptation, large and small, that comes my way. May you be glorified. Amen.

FROM THE DEVOTION ABOVE I HAVE IDENTIFIED . . .

The lie I believe:

The truth I now receive:

☐ ☐ ☐ I practiced healthy self-talk today (one to three times).

My key personal statement is:

☐ ☐ ☐ I have repeated that message at least three times today.

☐ I have written my personal statement above on an index card or in a journal that I can continue to read if I need renewal in this area.

Nourish Your Body—Tips from Losers

Everyone must discover what works best for them in the quest to get and stay lean for life. The following are tips that I have compiled from people who have lost weight and kept it off. You may find that some of their strategies work for you as well.

Tip #1: Always keep a healthy snack within reach. When you are hungry, it is difficult to resist the temptation of eating unhealthy foods that may be nearby. A healthy choice will help you stay on track and diminish the risk of consuming too many calories. Try out a variety of energy bars and find one you really enjoy. Put one ounce of your favorite nuts in ziplock bags. Keep an apple or banana in your purse or briefcase.

Tip #2: Record your successes. A journal allows you to validate your new commitment to health and wellness. The simple act of writing down each day's successes gives you a sense of accomplishment and new motivation. Have you started using this book's logging section each day? If not, try it today!

Tip #3: Practice portion control. In all my research, I notice that many people who finally realize permanent weight loss have perfected the skill of consistently reducing their portions. It is one of the simplest ways to change your lifestyle with very little thought or energy. When you can, take smaller amounts. When you are served large portions, save the rest for later whenever possible. When you can't do that . . . throw out the food and let go of the guilt.

Tip #4: Don't say "no," say "later." Those who adopt the attitude that they *can* eat anything they want but choose to delay that choice tend to indulge in empty calories less often and without the feeling of deprivation. And when they do indulge, they tend to eat less because they never say "never."

Tip #5: Give yourself grace. Don't beat yourself up if you overeat or miss getting exercise for a couple days. Shake it off and start fresh as soon as you can. Learning to cut your losses quickly is an important skill on the journey to living lean.

Tip #6: Practice good thinking. Call it whatever you will, healthy thinking is essential to all permanent change. Those who make lifestyle changes that stick have changed their old thinking patterns to new, empowering ones that move them in the right direction.

DAILY JOURNAL & LOG

My unhealthy habit(s) is diminishing and my new habits are increasing in the following ways:

Nutrition and Fat Management

I ate for maximum energy and health today in the following ways:

- ☐ By drinking 4 to 6 ounces of water most waking hours.
- ☐ By eating protein and/or fiber at breakfast.
- ☐ By eating 3 to 4 vegetables.
- ☐ By eating 2 to 3 servings of fruits, whole grains, or nuts.
- ☐ By eating 5 to 6 snacks or small meals.
- ☐ By eating less from bags and boxes.
- ☐ By eating only when I was hungry.
- ☐ By eating 20 to 50 percent less food than usual in the last 4 hours of the day.
- ☐ By eating no more than 10 percent "empty" calories.

Rest and Regeneration

Last night I slept ____________ hours.

The quality of my sleep was: _________________

Tonight I will ______________________________ to ensure I get quality rest.

Today I managed my stress by:

Tomorrow I will unwind and relax by:

☐ I practiced deep breathing today for relaxation and health.

Fitness

☐ Today I did my minimum 10 minutes of exercise.

I exceeded the minimum by _____________________

Tomorrow I will improve or maintain my fitness by:

Thoughts for Today

day 3

Nourish Your Spirit—Purified

> If we confess our sins, he is faithful and just and will forgive us our sins and purify us from all unrighteousness.
>
> 1 John 1:9

Pure fresh water flushes toxins out of our body and purifies it so all our organs can function optimally the way they were intended to function. If the water we drink is polluted, it can do just the opposite.

Confessing our sins to a holy God also purifies us. Jesus died for believers' sins: past, present, and future. If we are justified by his blood, forgiven, and going to heaven, why should we concern ourselves with confessing our sins? We need to confess and be purified "in time"—that is, right now—because our sin disrupts our fellowship with God and keeps us stuck. Yes, Jesus paid the price, but our behavior takes the confidence and power out of our walk with God. It also grieves the Holy Spirit who is in us (Eph. 4:30).

When young couples get married, they are usually idealist and cannot even imagine some of the challenges that lie ahead. They promise to love, honor, and cherish each other in good times and in bad. If they are serious about their covenant of marriage, they do not let disagreements, dishonesty, or even more grievous actions become grounds for divorce. But, no matter how unbreakable their commitment, they still need to work through their issues and restore the relationship to wholeness. Without confession (admitting one has wronged another through their actions) and repentance (turning from those actions and back to those that build up the marriage), the marriage is not fully alive.

In 1 John 1, the apostle of the same name recounts to believers all the wonderful truths about Jesus. He reminds us about the fellowship we have with God through Christ, so our joy will be complete. And then he shifts gears at the end of the chapter and starts to talk about sin. He tells us that if we say we have no sin, we are liars. But in the midst of that condemning blow, he gives us hope by telling us what to do with our day-to-day sins—confess them to a loving God. By doing so, we can know that we are purified from all unrighteousness and can walk once again in confident fellowship with the Lord.

Such a simple "formula" could be easily abused. If our God is so forgiving, then perhaps we can do whatever we want as long as we pray for forgiveness. If you look back to the marriage illustration, is that the kind of marriage you would want? Of course it isn't—and we don't want that kind of relationship with God either. His laws are perfect. They are designed to protect us and draw us close to him. Both in marriage and our fellowship with God, we want a relationship based on a covenant of love that always builds up. That is why our loving Father stands ready to forgive and restore us again and again. Shouldn't we do the same for each other?

Prayer

Oh Lord, how can I ever thank you for your loving-kindness to me? I pray that I will never take your forgiveness lightly. I will come to you immediately when I have sinned so I can be purified from all unrighteousness. Thank you for sending Jesus to die for my sins. Thank you for giving me the assurance I need that you forgive me day after day and restore me to complete fellowship with you. That restores my confidence and allows me to experience authentic intimacy with you. I love you, Lord. Amen.

FROM THE DEVOTION ABOVE I HAVE IDENTIFIED . . .

The lie I believe:

The truth I now receive:

☐ ☐ ☐ I practiced healthy self-talk today (one to three times).

My key personal statement is:

☐ ☐ ☐ I have repeated that message at least three times today.

☐ I have written my personal statement above on an index card or in a journal that I can continue to read if I need renewal in this area.

Nourish Your Body—Sugar Blues

We all know that sugar makes us gain weight and can cause cavities, and that overconsumption of it is a major factor in diabetes. But, if you are lean, brush your teeth after every meal, and aren't at high risk for diabetes, you may think you are safe. Well, you're not. Here are some sugar facts that could give you the sugar blues. Hopefully, they will motivate you to decrease your consumption and improve your health.

Beauty Blues

Many experts agree that eating too much sugar over a lifetime makes your skin more wrinkled and dull. The sugar in your blood attaches to proteins to form harmful new molecules called AGEs. The more sugar you eat, the more AGEs you develop. According to many skin experts, the most vulnerable cells in our body are collagen and elastin, both essential for maintaining young, supple skin. Amazingly, these aging effects can begin as early as age thirty-five and can increase exponentially unless the diet is changed. But it is never too late to reverse some of sugar's damaging effects. Obviously the first step is to cut back on sugar and other carbohydrates (such as packaged foods) that turn quickly to sugar in the body. For a little help on the outside, some of the skin care products that contain retinol can be very effective against wrinkles and dullness.

Energy Blues

Each time we eat easily digestible carbohydrates, our blood sugar goes up for a few minutes and then plummets lower than it was before we ate our treat. If we do that all day long, our energy goes down . . . down . . . down throughout the day. By evening all we want to do is eat and practice our couch potato skills. One rule I have followed fairly well for years is to avoid all sweets and low-fiber carbohydrates until late afternoon. Then, if I really want something sweet, I pick one thing and enjoy it fully.

Immunity Blues

The average person loses more than 90 percent of their immune function within fifteen minutes of indulging in sugar. This deficiency can last for up to two hours. Imagine what that means for people who put sugar in their coffee in the morning, eat a breakfast muffin at their morning break, include a cookie with lunch, eat a sugary snack in the late afternoon, and always have dessert after dinner. Those individuals could decrease their immunity for up to ten hours per day every day.

Cutting Back

The average American consumes 31 teaspoons per day of added sugar (sugar not naturally occurring in foods like fruits, vegetables, and grains). That equates to 465 sugar calories per day! As a point of reference, a 12-ounce soft drink has about 10 teaspoons of sugar. If you reduce your added sugar to no more than 10 teaspoons each day, you would consume only 150 calories of added sugar and greatly improve your health and vitality over time.

Your most dangerous form of sugar is high fructose corn syrup. This is a popular ingredient in soda pop and packaged foods. Read your labels and take small steps each day to reduce your sugar blues. You will increase your immunity and improve your skin tone in noticeable ways.

DAILY JOURNAL & LOG

My unhealthy habit(s) is diminishing and my new habits are increasing in the following ways:

Nutrition and Fat Management

I ate for maximum energy and health today in the following ways:

- ☐ By drinking 4 to 6 ounces of water most waking hours.
- ☐ By eating protein and/or fiber at breakfast.
- ☐ By eating 3 to 4 vegetables.
- ☐ By eating 2 to 3 servings of fruits, whole grains, or nuts.

☐ By eating 5 to 6 snacks or small meals.

☐ By eating less from bags and boxes.

☐ By eating only when I was hungry.

☐ By eating 20 to 50 percent less food than usual in the last 4 hours of the day.

☐ By eating no more than 10 percent "empty" calories.

Rest and Regeneration

Last night I slept ____________ hours.

The quality of my sleep was: _________________

Tonight I will ______________________________ to ensure I get quality rest.

Today I managed my stress by:

Tomorrow I will unwind and relax by:

☐ I practiced deep breathing today for relaxation and health.

Fitness

☐ Today I did my minimum 10 minutes of exercise.

I exceeded the minimum by _____________________

Tomorrow I will improve or maintain my fitness by:

Thoughts for Today

day 4

Nourish Your Spirit—Imitating God

> Be imitators of God, therefore, as dearly loved children and live a life of love, just as Christ loved us and gave himself up for us as a fragrant offering and sacrifice to God.
>
> Ephesians 5:1–2

My son invited two of his American friends from his school in Switzerland for a play date after school the other day. On the drive home, they started talking to each other in all the different accents they have been hearing the past two years attending an international school. I was amazed to hear French, Italian, German, British, and even Indian accents flowing from their mouths as they tried to make each other laugh with the silly comments they were making in their different personas. I was really surprised that my son, Jesse, could imitate his friends from Germany and England so well, to include their use of words like *rubbish* and *brilliant*.

People influence us greatly when we spend time with them every day. Good friends pick up each other's mannerisms and favorite words. They also can take on each other's bad habits. We become like the people we surround ourselves with. Without even realizing it, we often imitate them in both positive and negative ways. That's why we need to be purposeful about surrounding ourselves (and our children) with quality people.

Of course, no one is a perfect role model—that is, other than the Lord. That is why we are told to be "imitators of God." He is our model of love and sacrifice. When we imitate God, we practice giving ourselves up as an offering to others—sacrificing our time, gifts, and resources. The trendy little acronym WWJD (What Would Jesus Do?) is a helpful reminder to imitate Christ in the details of our lives. But we can't imitate Christ if we don't know him intimately and study his thoughts, words, and deeds.

Master impressionist Rich Little, who is famous for his impressions of many presidents and celebrities, says that it took him seven years to accurately mimic Frank Sinatra. But his dedication to his craft has transformed him from character to character on the stage where you no longer notice Rich but rather the person he is so impeccably mimicking at the moment.

Like Rich Little, we need to dedicate ourselves (no matter how long it takes) to the wonderful and transforming practice of imitating Christ. We can only do that as we observe him through the pages of Scripture and practice thinking, loving, and doing as he did. The reward of our imitation will not be fame or warm applause. But rather, our "audience of one" will be glorified as we become transformed into the very image of his Son.

Prayer

Heavenly Father, thank you for the perfect model of Christ. Help me to recall his life, words, and deeds as I go about my day. Forgive me for being influenced more by people than by you, and for sometimes being a poor role model to others. Teach me how to be a better imitator of Christ and to become transformed into his image. I pray this will be to your ultimate glory. Amen.

FROM THE DEVOTION ABOVE I HAVE IDENTIFIED . . .

The lie I believe:

The truth I now receive:

☐ ☐ ☐ I practiced healthy self-talk today (one to three times).

My key personal statement is:

☐ ☐ ☐ I have repeated that message at least three times today.

☐ I have written my personal statement above on an index card or in a journal that I can continue to read if I need renewal in this area.

Nourish Your Body—Forever Young

Did you know that we actually start aging on some levels at about age twenty-five to thirty years old? In the land of plenty, poor nutrition, increased pollution, and sedentary lifestyles are fast-forwarding many people's body clocks at an alarming rate. There are many factors influencing the rate at which we age. They include: (1) too much sugar and processed food; (2) too few antioxidant nutrients; (3) too much exposure to chemicals, pollutants, and heavy metals; (4) too little exercise; and (5) too much total food consumption. In fact, the only scientifically proven way to significantly extend your life (up to 30 percent) is to eat less food.

Of course, we need to eat to fuel our bodies. But every morsel that is not healthful and used for energy must be metabolized and excreted. Huge amounts of energy and bodily processes are used to accomplish this. It would be a useful exercise to stop ourselves before every single bite we take and ask, "Will this extend or shorten my life?" That may seem like an obsessive oversimplification, but it's really not. If we did just that most of the time (and acted on it healthfully), we'd be much healthier.

In the quest for good health and a long, vibrant life, we must realize that there is always a price to pay for every one of our choices. Investing in the amazing body God has given you for this short time on earth will significantly improve the journey. Listed below are some top antiaging supplements that may help you in that quest.

Anti-Aging Supplements

1. Super greens (rich in antioxidants and phytochemicals)
2. Quality vitamin-mineral supplement to fill in your nutritional gaps
3. Kyolic garlic (another powerful antioxidant and excellent immunity builder)
4. Omega-3 fish oils (for skin, brain, heart, and joints)
5. Green tea (super antioxidant and liver detoxifier)
6. Ginkgo biloba (improved mental function)
7. DHEA (this "antiaging" hormone should be taken only after hormone testing and under the direction of a health professional)

DAILY JOURNAL & LOG

My unhealthy habit(s) is diminishing and my new habits are increasing in the following ways:

Nutrition and Fat Management

I ate for maximum energy and health today in the following ways:

☐ By drinking 4 to 6 ounces of water most waking hours.

☐ By eating protein and/or fiber at breakfast.

☐ By eating 3 to 4 vegetables.

☐ By eating 2 to 3 servings of fruits, whole grains, or nuts.

☐ By eating 5 to 6 snacks or small meals.

☐ By eating less from bags and boxes.

☐ By eating only when I was hungry.

☐ By eating 20 to 50 percent less food than usual in the last 4 hours of the day.

☐ By eating no more than 10 percent "empty" calories.

Rest and Regeneration

Last night I slept ____________ hours.

The quality of my sleep was: _________________

Tonight I will ______________________________ to ensure I get quality rest.

Today I managed my stress by:

Tomorrow I will unwind and relax by:

☐ I practiced deep breathing today for relaxation and health.

Fitness

☐ Today I did my minimum 10 minutes of exercise.

I exceeded the minimum by _____________________

Tomorrow I will improve or maintain my fitness by:

Thoughts for Today

day 5

Nourish Your Spirit—Run for Cover

> Submit yourselves, then, to God. Resist the devil, and he will flee from you. Come near to God and he will come near to you.
>
> James 4:7–8

The old slogan for Lay's potato chips still plays in my mind on the rare occasion that I buy a bag of potato chips. "Betcha can't eat just one . . . betcha can't eat just one . . . betcha can't eat just one" chatters away in my brain until I fulfill its prophecy. The truth is, I *can* eat just one chip—I just don't.

Sometimes, our temptations come from a much more sinister source, the enemy himself—or more likely one of his workers. Being the "father of lies" (John 8:44), Satan knows that his best weapon is deception. If he can get us to believe a lie, his job is pretty much done, since most of us will act upon it without any influence once it is locked in to our minds. Sometimes we don't know if the lie is coming from our own unhealthy thoughts or from demonic sources. And it really doesn't matter. What does matter is how we respond at our first awareness of being tempted, distracted, or derailed.

James tells us to submit ourselves to God. But what does that mean? Submission in this day and age is often a word associated with being weak or "less than." The truth is we are weaker and "less than" almighty God. He calls us to submission to protect us. Running to God is like running for cover in a time of war. We don't stand out in the middle of a battle and let the bullets fly. Instead we hide in the safest place we can find.

Instead of bullets, we must be ready to take cover from the "flaming arrows of the evil one" (Eph. 6:16). He is trying to knock us off our stable foundation in Christ. But James tells us that if we submit to

God and resist the devil, he will actually flee from us. And then he reemphasizes the most important thing—staying near to God. God has allowed Satan some power for the time being, but his power will never come close to God's. When we draw near to God, our mighty Protector immediately meets us in our time of need. And when we are in his care, nothing can touch us—for greater is he who is in us, than he who is in the world (1 John 4:4).

The next time you feel tempted, run to God. The next time you are beating yourself up for your weaknesses or failures, run to God. The next time you feel confused and hopeless, run to God. Submit and surrender it all to the Lord and know in that moment that the enemy has run off with his tail between his legs.

Prayer

Dear Lord, you are my shelter from the temptations of life. You are my strength when the enemy is prowling about. Help me to surrender all my temptations, weaknesses, and failures to you, Father. Thank you for keeping me safe from the enemy. In Jesus's name, amen.

FROM THE DEVOTION ABOVE I HAVE IDENTIFIED . . .

The lie I believe:

The truth I now receive:

☐ ☐ ☐ I practiced healthy self-talk today (one to three times).

My key personal statement is:

☐ ☐ ☐ I have repeated that message at least three times today.

☐ I have written my personal statement above on an index card or in a journal that I can continue to read if I need renewal in this area.

Nourish Your Body—Ginkgo for Brainpower

While many factors contribute to a healthy brain, good circulation and nerve renewal top the list. The herb ginkgo biloba helps promote both. The leaves of the ginkgo, one of the oldest species of trees recorded, are the source for significant medicinal treatments that have been used for centuries all over the globe. Many researchers believe that ginkgo produces more antioxidant activity than many better-known antioxidants such as vitamins C, E, and beta-carotene. Several studies have shown that it exerts powerful antioxidant activity in the brain, eyes, and cardiovascular system. It is especially helpful in treating:

1. Memory loss
2. Attention deficit disorder (related to concentration, not hyperactivity)
3. Alzheimer's disease
4. Circulatory diseases
5. Depression
6. High blood pressure
7. Impotence
8. PMS
9. Radiation effects
10. Stroke
11. Vision problems

The recommended dosage ranges from 120 to 360 milligrams per day. It can take up to eight weeks for a therapeutic benefit to be realized.

Ginkgo protects blood vessels by reducing inflammation and can also be helpful in treating varicose veins. It is one of the best medicines in the world for improving circulation to the hands and feet. I'm so motivated, I'm going to go take my ginkgo right now!

DAILY JOURNAL & LOG

My unhealthy habit(s) is diminishing and my new habits are increasing in the following ways:

Nutrition and Fat Management

I ate for maximum energy and health today in the following ways:

- ☐ By drinking 4 to 6 ounces of water most waking hours.
- ☐ By eating protein and/or fiber at breakfast.
- ☐ By eating 3 to 4 vegetables.
- ☐ By eating 2 to 3 servings of fruits, whole grains, or nuts.
- ☐ By eating 5 to 6 snacks or small meals.
- ☐ By eating less from bags and boxes.
- ☐ By eating only when I was hungry.
- ☐ By eating 20 to 50 percent less food than usual in the last 4 hours of the day.
- ☐ By eating no more than 10 percent "empty" calories.

Rest and Regeneration

Last night I slept ____________ hours.

The quality of my sleep was: ________________

Tonight I will ______________________________ to ensure I get quality rest.

Today I managed my stress by:

Tomorrow I will unwind and relax by:

☐ I practiced deep breathing today for relaxation and health.

Fitness

☐ Today I did my minimum 10 minutes of exercise.

I exceeded the minimum by ____________________

Tomorrow I will improve or maintain my fitness by:

Thoughts for Today

day 6

Nourish Your Spirit—Worried and Upset

As Jesus and his disciples were on their way, he came to a village where a woman named Martha opened her home to him. She had a sister called Mary, who sat at the Lord's feet listening to what he said. But Martha was distracted by all the preparations that had to be made. She came to him and asked, "Lord, don't you care that my sister has left me to do the work by myself? Tell her to help me!"

> "Martha, Martha," the Lord answered, "*you are worried and upset about many things*, but only one thing is needed. Mary has chosen what is better, and it will not be taken away from her."
>
> Luke 10:38–42, emphasis added

I confess, I'm a type A woman, and in years past I often lived a totally out-of-balance life. I would pack my schedule so full of obligations and activities that I always felt stressed out. Fortunately, I finally realized that my persistent busyness was making me miss out on the best God had for me. Like Martha in the story above, I was "worried and upset about many things." And like Martha, I thought God was applauding my hard work.

When Martha asks Jesus in the passage above, "Lord, don't you care that my sister has left me to do the work by myself?" she doesn't even wait for him to answer! It seems that she actually assumes that he agrees with her, and then has the audacity to tell Jesus how to respond. She demands of him, "Tell her to help me!" Jesus couldn't even get a word in edgewise and must get Martha's attention by saying her name not once but twice—much like parents do with their children. Instead of agreeing with her, Jesus gives her a reality check and tells her what she cannot see: "You are worried and bothered about so many things."

When I first studied this, I felt that Jesus was rather harsh with Martha. And if I'd been her, my first reaction would have been to feel rejected. But the more I read this and processed it with an understanding of Jesus's pure and unconditional love, the more I realized that he loved Martha so much that he did not want her to miss the most important thing—the "one thing"—intimacy with him. Jesus did not say that Martha's activities were bad; he said that Mary's choice was better. And Jesus was willing to protect Mary from Martha's anger and frustration so that her worship and intimacy would not be diminished in any way. But as importantly, Jesus wanted Martha to experience the same for herself.

Are you letting busyness and expectations rob you from the "one thing"? Do pressures from others make you feel guilty when you try to get away by yourself and sit quietly at the Lord's feet? I know that I once did. But I won't let that lie influence me any longer. When I spend time with Christ, he fills me up, recenters my priorities, and gives me strength for the challenges of life. Without daily time with him, I am soon running on empty once again.

If you have never had consistent daily time with the Lord, let these daily readings and reflections be the start of a new spiritual habit. Except for illness or a spiritual fast, few of us get too busy to take in food for nourishment each day. We know that without it, we will soon be too hungry and fatigued to carry on. So, why do we try to run with our spiritual tanks on empty? I, like many of you, can be inconsistent in my quiet times with God. But, I want to crave my time with Jesus so much that I do everything in my power to steal intimate moments with him every chance I get . . . even when the "Martha" types are scurrying all around me!

Prayer

> Dear heavenly Father, thank you for loving us so much that you would put this story about Martha in your Word so we can clearly understand how much we miss when we put our busyness and plans ahead of you. Please help me to slow down and realize how much I am missing when I live this way. I love you, Lord. Please forgive me for not always making you the "one thing." Amen.

FROM THE DEVOTION ABOVE I HAVE IDENTIFIED . . .

The lie I believe:

The truth I now receive:

☐ ☐ ☐ I practiced healthy self-talk today (one to three times).

My key personal statement is:

☐ ☐ ☐ I have repeated that message at least three times today.

☐ I have written my personal statement above on an index card or in a journal that I can continue to read if I need renewal in this area.

Nourish Your Body—Rusting and Rotting

Our bodies are metabolic machines that turn oxygen into energy. In the process waste products called "free radicals" are formed. These substances are reactive and will wreak havoc in the cells of our body if they are not removed. In essence, they make our body both "rust and rot" on a continuous basis. What's the solution? Antioxidants!

These powerhouse nutrients clean up free radicals and carry them away from the body. Where damage has already occurred, they come in and correct the problem. Bestselling author Dr. James Balch explains in his book *The Super Anti-Oxidants* how a variety of antioxidant nutrients work in miraculous ways to protect us from a host of diseases. In fact, he says that there is one theory that almost all disease is an issue of a compromised immune system.[1] And a healthy immune system is dependent on a comprehensive and regular supply of antioxidants. How do we get those nutrients? Eat as many whole, natural foods as we can. Fruits, vegetables, whole grains, nuts, and seeds—foods the way God designed them; and supplement when necessary to fill in the gaps.

DAILY JOURNAL & LOG

My unhealthy habit(s) is diminishing and my new habits are increasing in the following ways:

Nutrition and Fat Management

I ate for maximum energy and health today in the following ways:

- ☐ By drinking 4 to 6 ounces of water most waking hours.
- ☐ By eating protein and/or fiber at breakfast.
- ☐ By eating 3 to 4 vegetables.
- ☐ By eating 2 to 3 servings of fruits, whole grains, or nuts.
- ☐ By eating 5 to 6 snacks or small meals.
- ☐ By eating less from bags and boxes.
- ☐ By eating only when I was hungry.
- ☐ By eating 20 to 50 percent less food than usual in the last 4 hours of the day.
- ☐ By eating no more than 10 percent "empty" calories.

Rest and Regeneration

Last night I slept ____________ hours.

The quality of my sleep was: _________________

Tonight I will ______________________________ to ensure I get quality rest.

Today I managed my stress by:

Tomorrow I will unwind and relax by:

☐ I practiced deep breathing today for relaxation and health.

Fitness

☐ Today I did my minimum 10 minutes of exercise.

I exceeded the minimum by ______________________

Tomorrow I will improve or maintain my fitness by:

Thoughts for Today

day 7

Nourish Your Spirit—Wearing God's Word

> Fix these words of mine in your hearts and minds; tie them as symbols on your hands and bind them on your foreheads. Teach them to your children, talking about them when you sit at home and when you walk along the road, when you lie down and when you get up.
>
> Deuteronomy 11:18–19

Can you imagine literally tying a small Bible onto your forehead and hands? Many Jews actually do something quite similar to that. They wear phylacteries (also called tefillin), which are small black leather boxes containing three key Torah passages that they believe God commanded adult males to literally bind to their bodies. During their daily prayer time, these men will strap on these boxes; one to the forehead and one to the "weak" arm in literal obedience. Our Scripture for today is a portion of one of those three passages. And, whether you believe that the Scripture above is literal or not, God was certainly making a powerful point. He wants us to be consumed by his Word. And not only as an individual but as a parent, talking about it constantly from sunrise to sunset. But does wearing God's Word really help us do that?

When I play tennis, I often wear a baseball cap. I am constantly aware of the brim as it shades my eyes from the sun and on occasion blocks my full vision of the ball. But even though I am noticing it is there, I rarely think about (or even remember) which hat I am wearing and what symbol or words everyone else can see. If I had an important Scripture on my hat, would I be influenced spiritually by wearing it every day? I suppose that depends on my perspective.

To me, the visual picture of a religious Jew wearing a tefellin on his forehead seems to say, "Lord, your Word is in the forefront of my mind. I will go to any length to show you how much I treasure it and love you for giving it to me." So, how can those of us who are not orthodox Jewish males respond to God's command to fix his Word in our hearts and minds?

If you eat only one meal per week, you will become weak and unable to perform even the simplest of daily activities. None of us would intentionally starve ourselves for months and years on end. But, many of us are starving spiritually. We need to consume the Word of God voraciously every day as if we had been starved without any food for days on end. To fix it in our minds, we need to think about it, memorize it, and pray about it constantly. God knows we are weak, and so he tells us with great detail what it will take to make it "stick" in a way that will consume our thoughts, influence our actions, and honor him.

Prayer

Father, please forgive me for not consistently being hungry for your Word. Help me to store it up in my heart and mind so that it transforms every part of my life. Please make me crave truth and fellowship with you more than anything else—so much that all I want to do is talk about you from sunrise to sunset. Amen.

FROM THE DEVOTION ABOVE I HAVE IDENTIFIED . . .

The lie I believe:

The truth I now receive:

☐ ☐ ☐ I practiced healthy self-talk today (one to three times).

My key personal statement is:

☐ ☐ ☐ I have repeated that message at least three times today.

☐ I have written my personal statement above on an index card or in a journal that I can continue to read if I need renewal in this area.

Nourish Your Body—Fitness Tips

You want your exercise sessions to count. The longer you exercise, the more calories you burn. And the more frequently you work out, the faster you improve your fitness. So, use a few of these tips to get more from your workouts.

1. Keeping your body temperature at a comfortable level will help you work out longer. Work out near a fan or on an exercise machine with a built-in fan. Wear cotton clothes that breathe. And always, always drink plenty of water before, during, and after exercise.
2. According to Heather Dillinger, an IDEA personal trainer, warming up for five minutes before each workout helps you lose more weight. It not only makes your muscles more pliable but also increases their range of motion, so you end up using more muscle fibers as you exercise.[1]
3. You can do crunches and sit-ups all day long, but the fat on top of the muscles is only going for a ride. It's important to get those muscles firm and conditioned, but for a lean waist and abdomen, you need to burn off the fat on top by doing regular aerobic exercise. The same goes for hips and thighs.
4. When you do the very same aerobic activity for months on end, your body becomes very efficient at it and over time will burn about 25 percent less calories. To maximize calorie burn, mix up your workouts by cross training. For example, walk one day, use a stationary bike the next, and perhaps take an exercise class at the gym or use a favorite exercise DVD.

DAILY JOURNAL & LOG

My unhealthy habit(s) is diminishing and my new habits are increasing in the following ways:

Nutrition and Fat Management

I ate for maximum energy and health today in the following ways:

- ☐ By drinking 4 to 6 ounces of water most waking hours.
- ☐ By eating protein and/or fiber at breakfast.
- ☐ By eating 3 to 4 vegetables.
- ☐ By eating 2 to 3 servings of fruits, whole grains, or nuts.
- ☐ By eating 5 to 6 snacks or small meals.
- ☐ By eating less from bags and boxes.
- ☐ By eating only when I was hungry.
- ☐ By eating 20 to 50 percent less food than usual in the last 4 hours of the day.
- ☐ By eating no more than 10 percent "empty" calories.

Rest and Regeneration

Last night I slept ____________ hours.

The quality of my sleep was: _________________

Tonight I will ______________________________ to ensure I get quality rest.

Today I managed my stress by:

Tomorrow I will unwind and relax by:

☐ I practiced deep breathing today for relaxation and health.

Fitness

☐ Today I did my minimum 10 minutes of exercise.

I exceeded the minimum by _____________________

Tomorrow I will improve or maintain my fitness by:

Thoughts for Today

day 8

Nourish Your Spirit—The Transformation

> But our citizenship is in heaven. And we eagerly await a Savior from there, the Lord Jesus Christ, who, by the power that enables him to bring everything under his control, will transform our lowly bodies so that they will be like his glorious body.
>
> Philippians 3:20

For the last two years, I have driven my son, Jesse, to the American School in Switzerland (TASIS) each morning. It is the only place in our temporary home of Lugano where he can get an education in English instead of Italian. TASIS is way too expensive for our income, but fortunately my husband's company was willing to foot the bill. As I drop him off each day, I see many of the children being driven to school by chauffeurs and nannies in limos. The moms and dads who do drive their children are dressed to the nines and driving a variety of expensive, exotic cars. Children here are indulged with all the best clothes, latest technology, and exotic vacations to some of the world's most expensive resorts. They have it all, and they do it all. When Jesse asked me for an iPhone because all his friends have them, I was relieved we'd be back in California for his sixth grade year! It has been quite a challenge to keep him grounded and not comparing our average lifestyle to those of his international friends.

God is so good in helping me show Jesse what is really important. Each day God allows us to experience a daily contrast to the life of excess at "the top of the hill" where TASIS is, to a very different scenario at the bottom of the hill. As we wait at the light both to and from school, Jesse and I watch a variety of handicapped children limp, hobble, and get pushed in wheelchairs into their special little school. None are driven by parents or chauffeurs, but nevertheless they are all smiling and laughing as they find their way on their own. Sometimes my heart breaks until I remember the verse above, which moves Jesse and me to pray that each of these children will come to know the Lord, so that their lowly bodies will one day be like Christ's glorious body. And if they do, we know in eternity that those children will be richer than the richest at the top of the hill because the power of the Savior who has everything under his control will raise them up to live in perfection for eternity!

Over time, like those children, our bodies also desire to be clothed in something perfect and imperishable. In our youth, in times of great health, in times of plenty, we embrace the blessings of life on earth. Yet, over the years, we lose our youthful appearance, watch our bodies slowly deteriorate, and sometimes even lose our material possessions. If we live long enough, we accept the reality that everything physical is temporary. Taking good care of our body is a form of worship to the Lord. Doing our part to stay healthy may extend our life and improve its quality. It is certainly worth the effort. Yet, even a perfect lifestyle will not halt the aging process or keep us from dying one day. It is such a great relief to know that no matter how much pain, disease, or struggles we face in this lifetime, one day we will have an absolutely perfect body in heaven. It is not something that money can buy; it is an amazing and excessive free gift lavished on those who are children of the King. And we all will live as heirs, not just at the top of some hill, but in the majesty of heaven!

Prayer

Heavenly Father, thank you for the hope of heaven. Just knowing that I will have a perfect, glorified body one day gives me great hope and peace. In the meantime, I pray that you will help me to be a good steward of the body you have given me for my time here on earth. In Jesus's name I pray, amen.

FROM THE DEVOTION ABOVE I HAVE IDENTIFIED . . .

The lie I believe:

The truth I now receive:

☐ ☐ ☐ I practiced healthy self-talk today (one to three times).

My key personal statement is:

☐ ☐ ☐ I have repeated that message at least three times today.

☐ I have written my personal statement above on an index card or in a journal that I can continue to read if I need renewal in this area.

Nourish Your Body—Fiber Facts for Energy and Health

Fiber is one of the most neglected elements of the American diet. The average person only eats about ten to fifteen grams per day. We need an absolute minimum of thirty grams. The best sources are fruits, vegetables, whole grains, and especially beans. An average serving contains about two to five grams. That means you would need about ten servings to meet your minimum requirement. Many cultures with diets that are high in fiber (up to fifty or more grams per day) have very low rates of heart disease and cancer. Fiber is essential for good health and has been linked to the prevention of many other diseases as well.

So what is fiber? It is the indigestible part of plant food. There are two kinds—soluble and insoluble. Think of the soluble fiber like a sponge that soaks up fluid and excess dietary fat as it travels through the digestive tract. Imagine the insoluble fiber like a scrub brush cleaning up the walls of your intestines as it travels the miles and miles of its journey.

Speaking of traveling, do you know how long it takes your food to travel from the time you eat it until its final exit? It should be about twelve to eighteen hours. That's called your transit time. A healthy transit time is important for general health and weight management. For good health, we don't want it to be too fast or too slow. If our transit time is sluggish, our food spends too much time in our digestive tract. Every single calorie is absorbed along with other toxins and unfavorable substances in our food.

I once heard a slow transit time compared with a big bowl of potato salad sitting in the sun on a picnic table. It builds up bacteria, has time to spoil, and loses its nutritional value. Ideally, we want a transit time that is healthy for adequate absorption of calories and other nutrients without undue exposure to the toxins in our foods like pesticides and additives. Soluble fiber does a great job attaching to dietary fat and carrying some of it out of the body. So, how do you test your transit time? It's very, very simple: eat some corn; look at your watch. Now, watch for the corn and look at your watch when it arrives! That's your transit time.

Fiber is not just for regularity. There is an important reason that it helps notch up your energy; it slows the release of carbohydrates into your bloodstream in the form of sugar. Let me give you an example. If you drink a glass of apple juice, the fructose (or natural fruit sugar) in the juice would quickly move into your bloodstream and your blood sugar would rise. That would give you an immediate boost of energy. But, the downside is that it also falls as quickly as it rose. Within a short period of time, your energy is waning. However, if you ate an apple instead of apple juice, the high fiber content in the apple slows down the release of the fruit sugars and your blood sugar rises more slowly and holds. Stabilize your blood sugar throughout the day by including fiber in every meal or snack. You will be amazed at the energy level over time. You will probably have less sugar cravings also.

DAILY JOURNAL & LOG

My unhealthy habit(s) is diminishing and my new habits are increasing in the following ways:

Nutrition and Fat Management

I ate for maximum energy and health today in the following ways:

- ☐ By drinking 4 to 6 ounces of water most waking hours.
- ☐ By eating protein and/or fiber at breakfast.
- ☐ By eating 3 to 4 vegetables.
- ☐ By eating 2 to 3 servings of fruits, whole grains, or nuts.
- ☐ By eating 5 to 6 snacks or small meals.
- ☐ By eating less from bags and boxes.
- ☐ By eating only when I was hungry.
- ☐ By eating 20 to 50 percent less food than usual in the last 4 hours of the day.
- ☐ By eating no more than 10 percent “empty” calories.

Rest and Regeneration

Last night I slept ____________ hours.

The quality of my sleep was: _________________

Tonight I will ______________________________ to ensure I get quality rest.

Today I managed my stress by:

Tomorrow I will unwind and relax by:

☐ I practiced deep breathing today for relaxation and health.

Fitness

☐ Today I did my minimum 10 minutes of exercise.

I exceeded the minimum by _____________________

Tomorrow I will improve or maintain my fitness by:

Thoughts for Today

day 9

Nourish Your Spirit—Mirror, Mirror

The LORD does not look at the things man looks at. Man looks at the outward appearance, but the LORD looks at the heart.

1 Samuel 16:7

As a young woman, I was terribly self-conscious about my appearance. Perhaps a more accurate word would be obsessed! I thought my thighs were excessively fat and that everyone noticed my "saddlebags." I wanted nothing more than to acquire the long, lean Barbie doll legs I had come to believe were the model of perfection. I was oblivious to the reality of my naturally narrow waist and flat stomach. All I saw were my fat legs. My perspective was totally warped and dishonoring to God.

Body image is just a part of our total self-image. However, in today's culture, how we look seems to have more significance than who we are. We are bombarded with magazine and television ads that seem to say we need to look a certain way. Beauty and our disproportionate attention to seeking the current "look" is really a matter of focus. One of the best things we can do to develop healthy body images is to change our focus. As they say, "Beauty is in the eye of the beholder." Will you behold society's image or God's? To behold God's image, you must refocus your attention on seeing yourself from God's viewpoint. He sees you as a complete person—body, soul, and spirit—and is most concerned about who you are inside. Yet, he doesn't want you to disregard your body either. Pray that he will give you an accurate perspective and a grateful spirit not only for who you are potentially but also exactly who you are this very moment. Reverse your negative thoughts about yourself and instead tell yourself the truth. For example:

God created me, and I am always beautiful in his eyes.
With God's help, I can have a healthy and reasonably lean body.
I celebrate my body and realize it is not the sum of who I am.
I can enjoy life without always thinking about how I look.
I am focusing on my strengths more than my perceived flaws.

You will never be content if you see yourself in comparison to others. The only person you need to strive to be like is Christ.

And, God is ready and willing to conform you to his image if you surrender to his model of perfection. Celebrate the unique person you were created to be! You are so much more than a physical body. Are you content to let God work through you to produce whatever results he pleases? Trust him to find the satisfaction you desire—a satisfaction that penetrates deeply beneath the surface to your very soul.

Prayer

Heavenly Father, I praise you for making me just who I am. Please forgive me for the times I have not taken good care of my body or when I have been discontent with how you chose to make me. Please help me to see myself through your eyes and to especially have a clean and humble heart, which is what you look on most. I love you, Lord. Amen.

FROM THE DEVOTION ABOVE I HAVE IDENTIFIED . . .

The lie I believe:

The truth I now receive:

☐ ☐ ☐ I practiced healthy self-talk today (one to three times).

My key personal statement is:

☐ ☐ ☐ I have repeated that message at least three times today.

☐ I have written my personal statement above on an index card or in a journal that I can continue to read if I need renewal in this area.

Nourish Your Body—Calorie-Counting Tips

As I said in chapter 4, counting calories is the most accurate way to honestly assess what you are eating if you need to lose weight and permanently change your eating habits. Even if you hate taking the time to do this, it will benefit you in huge ways. So with that in mind, here are a few tips.

Tip #1: Read the labels of already prepared foods like lasagna, pies, frozen entrees, or other prepackaged foods. It will give you an idea of what a serving size and calorie count might be on something you make at home or order in a restaurant.

Tip #2: Use index cards to write down the calorie content of the foods you eat most frequently. Try to prepare cards for at least two or three breakfast, lunch, and dinner options. Now you have a handy reference that's easy to use.

Tip #3: Become calorie "curious" without becoming calorie "obsessive." If it's too hard to figure out calories for a given snack or meal, just do portion control. Calorie counting does not have to be an all-or-nothing venture.

Tip #4: Challenge yourself to count calories for one month as if it were a business project that will produce a great bonus at the end. And it will. The bonus will be a loss of fat and gained insights into how to keep it off.

If I didn't convince you earlier of the importance of a reality check, let me reemphasize that now. This short-term exercise will have a profound effect on your choices for the rest of your life. Determine to take this short educational course in "calorie physics." Write down everything you eat and compute your calorie intake. Take on the attitude that if it's worth eating, it's worth writing down. You can look up and compute your calories as you go or you can calculate them at the end of the day.

The key to effective portion control and calorie counting is complete honesty. It is very easy to rationalize your own version of truth. Just keep reminding yourself that truth is not relative. Your body knows it; your fat cells reveal it! Being honest with yourself may seem like an enormous task at first. However, I guarantee that you will more clearly understand the role your choices are playing in changing your body. In no time, you will have a very clear concept of what you are really eating and burning. I have seen this exercise have a dramatic impact on the attitude and choices of many people.

Note: for many years, I have used my Caltrac Activity Monitor to give me an accurate assessment of my daily calorie burn. It also allows me to input my calories as I eat. It tells me if I am ahead of the game or behind by giving me the net excess or deficit of calories all day long. I've found this very helpful, and so have many of my clients.

DAILY JOURNAL & LOG

My unhealthy habit(s) is diminishing and my new habits are increasing in the following ways:

Nutrition and Fat Management

I ate for maximum energy and health today in the following ways:

- ☐ By drinking 4 to 6 ounces of water most waking hours.
- ☐ By eating protein and/or fiber at breakfast.
- ☐ By eating 3 to 4 vegetables.

- ☐ By eating 2 to 3 servings of fruits, whole grains, or nuts.
- ☐ By eating 5 to 6 snacks or small meals.
- ☐ By eating less from bags and boxes.
- ☐ By eating only when I was hungry.
- ☐ By eating 20 to 50 percent less food than usual in the last 4 hours of the day.
- ☐ By eating no more than 10 percent "empty" calories.

Rest and Regeneration

Last night I slept ____________ hours.

The quality of my sleep was: _________________

Tonight I will _______________________________ to ensure I get quality rest.

Today I managed my stress by:

Tomorrow I will unwind and relax by:

☐ I practiced deep breathing today for relaxation and health.

Fitness

☐ Today I did my minimum 10 minutes of exercise.

I exceeded the minimum by ______________________

Tomorrow I will improve or maintain my fitness by:

Thoughts for Today

day 10

Nourish Your Spirit—Body on Loan from God

> So whether you eat or drink or whatever you do, do it all for the glory of God.
>
> 1 Corinthians 10:31

The body God gave you may not fit in with the "dream" body the world says you must have to be accepted and valued. It may not run like a fine-tuned sports car. But, it is the only one you have. And if you see it through God's perspective and keep it fueled up and tuned up, it will serve you well.

It took me way too long to stop looking for shortcuts. I learned that there is a price to pay for a lean, healthy body. It is paid in the small details of your daily lifestyle. Oswald Chambers offers a pearl of wisdom when saying, "God will not give us good habits, He will not give us character, He will not make us walk aright. We have to do that for ourselves. Beware of the tendency of asking the way when you know it perfectly well."[1]

Each day as you make choices about what to eat, drink, or act upon, try to keep God's glorification always before your personal gratification. Unless we make a constant and conscious effort to seek first the kingdom of God and his righteousness, chances are that our needs and wants will always float to the top.

God has provided all we need to reach our best potential—whatever he has ordained that to be. He has given us food to eat, air to breathe, water to drink, and his Word to completely satiate our souls and spirits. If we think about the quality of his original resources, they were perfect. Unfortunately, we humans have a tendency to pollute and destroy God's best. If we simply go back to the basics in all areas—natural food, pure fresh water, clean air, and the unadulterated Word of God—we would be absolutely amazed at what we can "grow" . . . a healthier body, soul, and spirit!

Prayer

Dear Lord, thank you for providing me with all I need to be my best. Please forgive me for too often seeking my own gratification first. I pray your Holy Spirit will prompt me when I am doing that and remind me of my heart's desire to glorify you in all I do. Teach me and guide me as I am often weak and self-centered. I pray you will grow me into the person you created me to be. In Jesus's name I pray, amen.

FROM THE DEVOTION ABOVE I HAVE IDENTIFIED . . .

The lie I believe:

The truth I now receive:

☐ ☐ ☐ I practiced healthy self-talk today (one to three times).

My key personal statement is:

☐ ☐ ☐ I have repeated that message at least three times today.

☐ I have written my personal statement above on an index card or in a journal that I can continue to read if I need renewal in this area.

Nourish Your Body—Conquering Cellulite

Cellulite is the lumpy, bumpy fat that tends to accumulate in the thighs, hips, and buttocks of many women of all shapes and sizes. While gender and genetics influence your predisposition to cellulite formation, lifestyle plays a much more important role. You can diminish the appearance of cottage cheese–like fat on the backside of your body by consistently implementing the following habits (many of which have been already discussed related to a healthy lifestyle).

Deflate overstuffed fat cells. As an adult, you have all the fat cells you will ever get (twenty to sixty billion). However, they have an almost unlimited capacity to fill. Do not focus on weight on the scale. Focus on accessing and burning stored fat. Do not diet! Diets often burn stored carbohydrate and muscle. If you consistently burn more calories than you eat in a way that supports your metabolism, chances are the weight you lose will be fat.

Eat and burn all day long. Your body actually knows about how many calories it needs at specific times of day. And if you don't fuel up right, it revolts . . . with fatigue, cravings, and more efficient fat storage. By eating and burning all day long with more frequent yet small meals or snacks, your body knows it will have sufficient immediate fuel to get through the day. So get lean and energized by eating most of your calories in the first twelve hours of your day when you burn them best!

Increase your circulation. Cellulite forms in areas of the body regulated by a body pump called the lymphatic system. To keep nutrients and waste products flowing in and out, it requires stimulation from muscular contractions. The more you move, the better it pumps. So get up and get going! Don't invest in expensive creams and potions. In addition to regular exercise, vigorous massage with body lotion after your shower can improve blood flow to trouble spots and help remove toxins. Don't expect miracles, however.

Drink ten to twelve glasses of water every day. A good rule of thumb is to drink four to eight ounces of water for every hour you're awake. The human body is 60–70 percent water. Every bodily function occurs in a medium of water. Our body needs plenty of water to rid itself of the waste products of metabolism. The cells get congested in the areas of poorest circulation. To diminish toxic buildup, drink up and avoid carbonated beverages, as they actually increase the congestion.

Increase your potassium intake. The lumpy, bumpy look of cellulite appears in areas where the fluid between cells is congested and edematous due to a sodium/potassium imbalance. Your body needs twice as much potassium as sodium. But most people eat just the opposite. Eat lots of fruits and vegetables (which are ten to one hundred times higher in potassium than sodium). Decrease your salt intake, and soon you will see a smoother "backside"!

DAILY JOURNAL & LOG

My unhealthy habit(s) is diminishing and my new habits are increasing in the following ways:

Nutrition and Fat Management

I ate for maximum energy and health today in the following ways:

- ☐ By drinking 4 to 6 ounces of water most waking hours.
- ☐ By eating protein and/or fiber at breakfast.
- ☐ By eating 3 to 4 vegetables.
- ☐ By eating 2 to 3 servings of fruits, whole grains, or nuts.
- ☐ By eating 5 to 6 snacks or small meals.
- ☐ By eating less from bags and boxes.
- ☐ By eating only when I was hungry.

☐ By eating 20 to 50 percent less food than usual in the last 4 hours of the day.

☐ By eating no more than 10 percent "empty" calories.

Rest and Regeneration

Last night I slept ___________ hours.

The quality of my sleep was: ________________

Tonight I will ____________________________ to ensure I get quality rest.

Today I managed my stress by:

Tomorrow I will unwind and relax by:

☐ I practiced deep breathing today for relaxation and health.

Fitness

☐ Today I did my minimum 10 minutes of exercise.

I exceeded the minimum by ____________________

Tomorrow I will improve or maintain my fitness by:

Thoughts for Today

day 11

Nourish Your Spirit—The Beginning of Wisdom

> The fear of the LORD is the beginning of wisdom, and knowledge of the Holy One is understanding.
>
> Proverbs 9:10

Fear is a terrifying emotion. How's that for an obvious statement! Most of us avoid it at almost any cost. We flee from that which we fear. If you fear heights, you stay away from the edge. If you fear large dogs, you cross the street when you see one approaching. If you fear being rejected, you avoid intimacy.

Yet fearing God is different. We are to draw near to the very one we are told to fear.

Those of us who have a saving faith in Jesus Christ have been pardoned from all our sins and can now approach the throne of grace with confidence (Heb. 4:16). Does our salvation negate our need to fear God? Apparently not, as Luke writes in Acts 9:31: "Then the church throughout Judea, Galilee and Samaria enjoyed a time of peace. It was strengthened; and encouraged by the Holy Spirit, it grew in numbers, living in the fear of the Lord."

The fear of God in the life of the believer is part reverence and awe and part trembling and quaking as we consider the immensity and omnipotence of the God we love and serve. If we take his incredible grace for granted and believe we no longer need to fear him, we are mistaken. While the blood of Christ has cleansed us from all sin and secured our place in heaven, we must live knowing that the God who loves us enough to send his one and only Son to die for us will also discipline us as he molds us into the image of Christ.

When we have a healthy fear of the Lord balanced with a great confidence that comes from his mercy and grace found only in Christ, we have the beginning of wisdom. And as we come to know him through his Word and prayer, our understanding grows.

Abraham Lincoln said, "I have been driven many times to my knees by the overwhelming conviction that I had no where else to go. My own wisdom, and that of all about me, seemed insufficient for the day."[1] Realizing our insufficiency and "fearing the Lord" allows us to be open to his teaching and divine guidance. Those who think they have all the answers are often tripped up by their own arrogance and self-sufficiency. Fear of the Lord requires a humble, open spirit that constantly acknowledges God's sovereignty and total wisdom. It is in that state of fear and awe that God can use us most profoundly.

Wisdom and understanding come to a heart that has a healthy fear of God and is committed to applying his precepts. Corrie Ten Boom said, "Don't worry about what you do not yet understand . . . worry about what you do understand but do not live by."[2]

Prayer

Dear Lord, you are all-powerful, all-knowing, all-encompassing. You are mighty to be feared. Forgive me when I have taken your mercy and grace for granted and have not given you the reverence and fear you so deserve. I bow my heart in awe of you today and pray your forgiveness for my arrogance. You alone are God. You alone are worthy to be praised. I will love and fear you all the days of my life. Thank you for extending your mercy and grace to me—once a sinner—now a saint! In Jesus's name, amen.

FROM THE DEVOTION ABOVE I HAVE IDENTIFIED . . .

The lie I believe:

The truth I now receive:

☐ ☐ ☐ I practiced healthy self-talk today (one to three times).

My key personal statement is:

☐ ☐ ☐ I have repeated that message at least three times today.

☐ I have written my personal statement above on an index card or in a journal that I can continue to read if I need renewal in this area.

Nourish Your Body—The Brain-Beauty Connection

"Gee, you look so young for your age. What's your beauty secret?"

Wouldn't you love to be asked that question? You may be surprised to know the secret is not the latest, greatest skin care product. It is a powerful nutrient that stimulates your brain, revitalizes your skin, slows down aging, improves fat metabolism, lubricates your joints, decreases inflammation, and protects your heart. The problem is that this "mystery" nutrient is found in only a handful of foods that you rarely eat on a daily basis. If you don't address this nutritional gap, your body and, most importantly, your brain will be short-changed. The nutrient I am talking about is an essential fatty acid called omega-3. It is one of only two fats that are considered essential for life, the other being omega-6. Our body cannot produce these fats and must have them to function properly. I've been notching up my omegas for about eight years, and I can see the big difference in my skin. At fifty-five, I am often mistaken for a woman in her midforties.

And, except for my occasional hormonal "menopause brain freezes," my ability to concentrate and recall information is terrific!

Younger Inside and Out

Because brain cells are largely composed of fat, the right kind of fat in the diet is the most critical element in creating and maintaining brain health. The skin (your largest organ of your body) requires the exact same nutrients to stay young or even reverse the signs of aging. Omega-3 fatty acids are the single most important nutrient that feeds our brain and skin! With good omega-3 nutrition, both are healthy and well nourished. Each cell is plumped up like a ripe grape, smooth and firm instead of shriveled up like a raisin. We can spend a fortune on creams and makeup, but nothing takes the place of skin care from the inside out!

Are You Getting Enough Omega-3 Fat?

The best sources of omega-3 essential fatty acids are salmon, swordfish, tuna, shark, pecans, almonds, walnuts, soy nuts, flaxseed, and deep green vegetables like kale and turnip greens. So, let me ask you a question. How many of these foods do you eat every day? We need the equivalent amount of omega-3 fats we find in a serving of salmon (about 3,500 milligrams) every day. All the other sources (even fish) are at least one-quarter the amount found in salmon specifically. Sadly, if we eat enough fish to meet our daily need for omega-3 fat, we'd be glowing in the dark from heavy metal contamination—just one more sad example of man's lack of stewardship for the resources God has so abundantly provided.

Therefore, supplementation is essential. Since not all supplements are equal and omega-3 fats can spoil quickly, I did some research and recommend the Ultimate Omegas by Nordic Naturals and Coromega. Both are excellent products that I use personally and carry on my website for those who cannot find them in their local health food stores.

There is much more to say about this essential and powerful nutrient, so we will expand on this tomorrow.

DAILY JOURNAL & LOG

My unhealthy habit(s) is diminishing and my new habits are increasing in the following ways:

Nutrition and Fat Management

I ate for maximum energy and health today in the following ways:

- ☐ By drinking 4 to 6 ounces of water most waking hours.
- ☐ By eating protein and/or fiber at breakfast.
- ☐ By eating 3 to 4 vegetables.
- ☐ By eating 2 to 3 servings of fruits, whole grains, or nuts.
- ☐ By eating 5 to 6 snacks or small meals.
- ☐ By eating less from bags and boxes.
- ☐ By eating only when I was hungry.
- ☐ By eating 20 to 50 percent less food than usual in the last 4 hours of the day.
- ☐ By eating no more than 10 percent "empty" calories.

Rest and Regeneration

Last night I slept ____________ hours.

The quality of my sleep was: ________________

Tonight I will ______________________________ to ensure I get quality rest.

Today I managed my stress by:

Tomorrow I will unwind and relax by:

☐ I practiced deep breathing today for relaxation and health.

Fitness

☐ Today I did my minimum 10 minutes of exercise.

I exceeded the minimum by ____________________

Tomorrow I will improve or maintain my fitness by:

Thoughts for Today

day 12

Nourish Your Spirit—The Ticket

> Your word is a lamp to my feet
> and a light for my path.
> I have taken an oath and confirmed it,
> that I will follow your righteous laws.
>
> Psalm 119:105–106

God's laws are good for us. Most of us know that and yet we cut corners and make up our own rules as if our wisdom surpasses God's. We eat to please our palate more than nourish our cells. We spend money on what we want more often than on what we need. We do all sorts of things that break what we would call "little rules" while always keeping the big ones. We'd never rob a bank, but do we handle our money according to God's Word? We'd never harm someone intentionally, but do we break God's heart by lacking compassion or a willingness to give to those less fortunate than us? In little ways we mold God's and man's rules to suit our own needs.

The reality of my own disobedience really hit me the other day when I read about a man named Jack who had been pulled over (once again) for speeding. He was going about fifty-five miles per hour in a thirty zone when he was caught. To his dismay, the police officer was an acquaintance from his prayer group at church. Needless to say, he was embarrassed, but that didn't stop him from trying to get out of his ticket and hoping his casual relationship would help his cause. Despite his efforts at levity and good excuses, the officer remained very stern. Jack waited and waited for his ticket. Finally the officer returned to his car and handed him a folded piece of paper with the admonishment, "Slow down, Jack." Jack sat there with the paper in his hand as the patrol car rolled away. He opened it slowly, expecting a hefty fine. It read:

> Dear Jack, once upon a time I had a daughter. She was six when she was killed by a car. You guessed it—a speeding driver. A fine and three months in jail, and the man was free . . . free to hug his daughters, all three of them. I only had one, and I'm going to have to wait until heaven before I can ever hug her again. A thousand times I've tried to forgive that man. A thousand times I thought I had. Maybe I did, but I need to do it again. Pray for me. And be careful. My son is all I have left.
>
> Signed, Bob

God gives us boundaries—not to restrict our freedom but to protect us (and others) from harm. Even when we think breaking a little rule will do no harm, we really don't know the future. I have read verse 105 above hundreds of times over the years, but I never really spent time on verse 106. Perhaps that is our problem; just as we pick and choose the precepts we will follow, we pick and choose the Scriptures we study. What good is it to acknowledge that God's Word is a light to our path if we are unwilling to follow it? Today, I am going to make an oath and confirm it with someone close to me: that I will follow God's righteous laws to my best ability. I know I will stumble and fall. I know only by God's power and grace can I be faithful. If we are willing, God will not only illuminate our path so we can walk in righteousness, he will give us great joy in the walk.

Prayer

Oh Lord, thank you for the power and truth in your Word. Thank you for loving us so much that you would want to show us the way to walk. Yet, it is so hard sometimes. Please forgive me for choosing my way too often. I pray that you show me in your Word how to live in the areas of my life that I struggle with most. I know your Word is living and active, and I ask that you allow it to cut the lies and rebellion out of me and replace it with passion for seeking you alone. Thank you for your mercy and forgiveness. Thank you for loving me despite my failure. In Jesus's name, amen.

FROM THE DEVOTION ABOVE I HAVE IDENTIFIED . . .

The lie I believe:

The truth I now receive:

☐ ☐ ☐ I practiced healthy self-talk today (one to three times).

My key personal statement is:

☐ ☐ ☐ I have repeated that message at least three times today.

☐ I have written my personal statement above on an index card or in a journal that I can continue to read if I need renewal in this area.

Nourish Your Body—More Fat Facts

If having healthier skin and brain cells did not motivate you enough to increase your intake of omega-3 fats, perhaps today's teaching will. According to Dr. Jordan Rubin, author of *The Maker's Diet*, "There may not be a single nutritional supplement or pharmacological drug today that can offer the same level of protection against cancer, heart disease, and the inflammatory response that impacts many other diseases."[1]

The balance of the two essential fatty acids (omega-3 and omega-6) is critical to good health. Omega-6 fatty acids are found in vegetable oils. They are very easy to get into our diets on a daily basis because the food industry made a massive shift away from using animal fats, such as butter and lard, to making products out of vegetable fats. Commercial baked goods, salad dressings, and cooking oils are all based on these plant source fats, like soybean and canola oil. Yes, they are much better for us than the alternative. But, you can get too much of a good thing. As a result of this shift, most people are getting too many omega-6 fatty acids while getting way too little omega-3. This has created an unhealthy disparity, and the imbalance causes an inflammatory response all over our bodies, hardening areas of the brain, creating cardiovascular disease, decreasing lubrication in our joints, and aging our skin and more.

While the ideal ratio of omega-3 to omega-6 should be somewhere between 1:1 and 1:3, the majority of Americans are at ratios of 1:20 to 1:30. This huge discrepancy is causing significant health concerns. Since most people get sufficient omega-6 fatty acids in their diet, the practical challenge is to eat less omega-6 and many more of the omega-3 fatty acids. Try cooking with olive oil as it is an omega-9 fatty acid and will not contribute to an unhealthy fat ratio.

Poor lifestyle and diet, ongoing stress, smoking, and environmental pollutants all damage fragile brain cells and damage our skin cells, causing wrinkles and premature aging. People who abuse their bodies through poor diet and lifestyle can experience mental falloff as early as their thirties, including mood swings.

Many compelling studies are revealing that omega-3 supplementation decreases aggressive behavior, diminishes depression, protects against Alzheimer's disease, and fosters mental clarity. Just imagine your brain as healthy, well nourished, and firing on all eight cylinders as opposed to being clogged up, bogged down, and blowing its fuses because it has been poorly fed with artificial sweeteners and unhealthy fats. Pure, fresh water and sufficient omega-3 fats provide the ultimate nutrients for a responsive brain and glowing skin.

So, are you motivated now to eat more omega-3 rich foods and add daily supplementation into your lifestyle? Your body will love you if you do.

DAILY JOURNAL & LOG

My unhealthy habit(s) is diminishing and my new habits are increasing in the following ways:

Nutrition and Fat Management

I ate for maximum energy and health today in the following ways:

- ☐ By drinking 4 to 6 ounces of water most waking hours.
- ☐ By eating protein and/or fiber at breakfast.
- ☐ By eating 3 to 4 vegetables.
- ☐ By eating 2 to 3 servings of fruits, whole grains, or nuts.
- ☐ By eating 5 to 6 snacks or small meals.
- ☐ By eating less from bags and boxes.
- ☐ By eating only when I was hungry.
- ☐ By eating 20 to 50 percent less food than usual in the last 4 hours of the day.
- ☐ By eating no more than 10 percent "empty" calories.

Rest and Regeneration

Last night I slept ____________ hours.

The quality of my sleep was: ________________

Tonight I will ______________________________ to ensure I get quality rest.

Today I managed my stress by:

Tomorrow I will unwind and relax by:

☐ I practiced deep breathing today for relaxation and health.

Fitness

☐ Today I did my minimum 10 minutes of exercise.

I exceeded the minimum by ____________________

Tomorrow I will improve or maintain my fitness by:

Thoughts for Today

day 13

Nourish Your Spirit—The Abundant Life

> I have come that they may have life, and have it to the full.
>
> John 10:10

The word *abundant* conjures up thoughts of something overflowing in sufficiency. If we have abundant health, we have more vitality and energy than we can possibly use. If we have abundant wealth, we cannot outspend or outgive our resources. If we have abundant relationships, our life is overflowing with people who know and love us. As humans, we want abundant lives . . . we crave them. As Christians we actually already have them. But we sometimes miss the value of the treasures God has stored up for those who love him.

> "No eye has seen, no ear has heard, no mind has conceived what God has prepared for those who love him"—but God has revealed it to us by his Spirit.
>
> 1 Corinthians 2:9

The moment we come to believe that Jesus is truly the only way to be saved and have intimacy with the living God, we become coheirs with him for all eternity. We have all we need to live complete, joyful, and purposeful lives. Yet, our "abundant life" does not look like the life that our culture would have you believe we need to be happy. Today, fame, fortune, beauty, and power are the things most people crave. They crave them only because the holes in their hearts are not yet filled with Christ's abundance. They know no other way.

But what about those of us who know Christ yet are not celebrating the abundance he promises? It seems too many are saved without victory—victory to live abundantly despite their circumstances. How can this be? It is because their focus is on the values of the world (that world we are told *not* to conform to in Romans 12:2) rather than on renewing their minds and worshipping God for all he has provided.

For two years, I have lived in one of the wealthiest areas of the world, Lugano, Switzerland. It is a place rich with beauty in the foothills of the Alps. And it is a place full of extremely rich people. It is not uncommon for some to spend hundreds of thousands of dollars on their cars. Women wear the largest diamonds I've ever seen on their ears, on their hands, around their necks, and in their belly buttons! They shop until they drop, worshipping Gucci and Prada. They have an abundance of things and yet seem so very empty.

We drive our Honda Jazz, wear our Levis jeans, and eat pizza in the little restaurants because we cannot justify spending over three hundred francs on dinner for two. It has been hard just to pay our sky-high gasoline and utility bills. And yet, my husband, Lew, and I know that our simple little life is so much more abundant than the richest of the rich here in Lugano. If only they knew our Jesus, they could be truly rich also and know what Jesus meant when he said, "I came that they might have life and have it abundantly."

Prayer

Dear Lord, I know in my mind that you have already given me all I need to live a truly abundant life. Please help me to remember this when I get distracted by the world and its values. I love you and want to honor you with a heart of contentment. In Jesus's name, amen.

FROM THE DEVOTION ABOVE I HAVE IDENTIFIED . . .

The lie I believe:

The truth I now receive:

☐ ☐ ☐ I practiced healthy self-talk today (one to three times).

My key personal statement is:

☐ ☐ ☐ I have repeated that message at least three times today.

☐ I have written my personal statement above on an index card or in a journal that I can continue to read if I need renewal in this area.

Nourish Your Body—Growing Healthy Families

While some of you may not have spouses or children at this time, you may one day. And many of us have close connections with our nieces, nephews, and friends' children. So, I hope you will embrace this teaching on behalf of any children you have (or will have) in your life.

Parents and children both have their own unique responsibilities when it comes to mealtime. A child's responsibility is to chew and swallow. The parent's responsibility is to provide a variety of healthy foods in a relaxed environment. When these lines are crossed or confused, mealtimes can become very unpleasant. It is important for parents, grandparents, and caretakers to realize that every eating experience is an adventure for your child. Many skills are required for young children to master eating, from grasping a fork to capturing a roll-away pea, not to mention simply getting something slippery or a little scary-looking into their mouths and ultimately swallowed. And young children engage most of their senses (smell, touch, sight, and taste . . . sometimes even sound) when they are discovering and eating foods. They love to feel it squishy or crunchy in their little hands and often will play with it before it enters their mouths. Of course, we should accept that of our twelve- to twenty-four-month child. When a child is six years old, food experiments at the dinner table are unacceptable.

As adults, we need to slow down and approach mealtime with the same wonder, amazement, and sometimes fright that the child experiences—realizing that it takes at least eight exposures to a new food before a child can actually develop a positive "taste" for that food—no matter how old they may be! The taste buds actually grow and mature as they are exposed to a variety of new tastes and textures. Unfortunately, most parents give up after one or two negative experiences, throwing up their hands and exclaiming, "Johnny just hates vegetables." But the truth is that Johnny never really got a chance to develop a taste for those veggies. Mom or Dad caved in to his initial negative response, and Johnny is ultimately the loser as his little body is shortchanged by not receiving all the incredible nutrients God power-packed into many healthy foods.

It is essential that as parents we realize that we are laying a nutritional foundation for our children that will impact them for a lifetime. If we get lazy and follow the course of least resistance by caving in every time they respond negatively, or if we live such a busy lifestyle that we visit fast-food restaurants more than grocery stores, our children will inherit poor attitudes and habits that will impact their health and wellness for decades. On the other hand, we don't have to be food Nazis either. Find the balance between excellent nutrition and practical enjoyment of food. Start wherever you are in the nutritional spectrum and slowly notch up the quality and consistency of healthy foods a little each week. You will be amazed over the course of a year how much your family's nutrition can change, and they may not even miss all the junk foods that have slowly disappeared from your fridge and pantry.

DAILY JOURNAL & LOG

My unhealthy habit(s) is diminishing and my new habits are increasing in the following ways:

Nutrition and Fat Management

I ate for maximum energy and health today in the following ways:

- ☐ By drinking 4 to 6 ounces of water most waking hours.
- ☐ By eating protein and/or fiber at breakfast.
- ☐ By eating 3 to 4 vegetables.
- ☐ By eating 2 to 3 servings of fruits, whole grains, or nuts.
- ☐ By eating 5 to 6 snacks or small meals.
- ☐ By eating less from bags and boxes.
- ☐ By eating only when I was hungry.
- ☐ By eating 20 to 50 percent less food than usual in the last 4 hours of the day.
- ☐ By eating no more than 10 percent "empty" calories.

Rest and Regeneration

Last night I slept ____________ hours.

The quality of my sleep was: _________________

Tonight I will ______________________________ to ensure I get quality rest.

Today I managed my stress by:

Tomorrow I will unwind and relax by:

☐ I practiced deep breathing today for relaxation and health.

Fitness

☐ Today I did my minimum 10 minutes of exercise.

I exceeded the minimum by ____________________

Tomorrow I will improve or maintain my fitness by:

Thoughts for Today

day 14

Nourish Your Spirit—Rich in the Word

> Let the word of Christ dwell in you richly as you teach and admonish one another with all wisdom, and as you sing psalms, hymns and spiritual songs with gratitude in your hearts to God. And whatever you do, whether in word or deed, do it all in the name of the Lord Jesus, giving thanks to God the Father through him.
>
> Colossians 3:16–17

Have you ever met someone who is so enamored by another person that they can't stop talking about them? In some cases, it may be a business guru whose teaching has been instrumental to another's success, and as a result that expert becomes the source of instruction whenever an important decision or action is undertaken. "Mr. Smith says this" or "Mr. Smith does that" seems to precede many comments. It is obvious that Mr. Smith's words are richly dwelling in this person's mind.

God wants his words to dwell in us above any other, so much so that it influences everything we do. For that to happen, we must take the time to put his truth into our minds through study and meditation. And over time, it will migrate to our hearts. The Word of Christ is not something that happens without considerable effort. God has given us so much to read and ponder in his personal love letter to us—the Bible. But once the truth of Scripture is resident in our hearts, it can overflow to others, teaching and encouraging them with wisdom. It also is essential that God's truth be the center of our worship. If we exalt God with words and songs that do not honor him, we actually dishonor him. Gratitude then becomes a natural outflow of a heart that is abundantly full of truth from Scripture.

Like the healthy habits of mind and body we are trying to establish, healthy spiritual habits are essential to our well-being. And just as accurate thinking transforms our bodily habits, accurate thinking about God transforms our spiritual habits. If we are to do everything in the name of the Lord Jesus as it says above, that will be impossible if we don't know truth. It says in Psalm 119:11: "I have hidden your word in my heart that I might not sin against you." It is the Word of God animated by the Holy Spirit that allows our words and deeds to glorify the Lord.

Just as we need daily food and water to survive physically, we need to consume the Word of God to survive spiritually. There are limits to how much food we can or should eat. But, we can never ingest too much truth. God doesn't want us to merely survive. He wants us to be filled to overflowing so that we cannot even begin to hold in the love, joy, and hope only his truth can give—so full we must sing his praises to the heavens.

Prayer

Father in heaven, I know that your Word is truth. It reveals who you are and shows me how to live victoriously. It teaches me and molds me. Forgive me when I spend more time seeking worldly knowledge than knowledge about you. Help me to crave your Word, Lord, and feel ravenous in my spirit for your truth. Amen.

FROM THE DEVOTION ABOVE I HAVE IDENTIFIED . . .

The lie I believe:

The truth I now receive:

☐ ☐ ☐ I practiced healthy self-talk today (one to three times).

My key personal statement is:

☐ ☐ ☐ I have repeated that message at least three times today.

☐ I have written my personal statement above on an index card or in a journal that I can continue to read if I need renewal in this area.

Nourish Your Body—Health Tidbits You Can Use

Mega Portions

More often than not, portions you receive in restaurants are two to four times larger than most nutritionists recommend as healthy servings. Don't feel you must eat everything served to you. Either share a meal with a friend or take the leftovers home with you for another meal. That saves calories and money.

Chew, Chew, Chew

Chewing veggies well helps release chemicals that are known to help your body in the production and regulation of white blood cells—your natural infection-fighting warriors. In his book *The Great Physician's Rx for Health and Wellness*, author Jordan Rubin writes, "Chewing slowly and thoroughly can also help maintain a healthy weight as you allow your brain to register the amount of food you are consuming. Put simply, people who chew more consciously, eat less."[1]

It's the Small Stuff

By simply choosing an open-face sandwich (one slice of bread), you can save 100–120 calories at lunchtime. Switch out fried chips for baked and you save another 50–75 calories. Drink water instead of juice or soda . . . another 150, for a total of 300–345. Make those kind of small changes every day, and you'll be 30 pounds lighter in a year!

Eat Fish . . . but Be Wise

Fish is a great source of omega-3 fatty acids and protein, but sadly some are more contaminated than others with PCBs (industrial chemicals). Wild Alaskan salmon is a better choice than farmed salmon. Some experts say that striped bass is always very high in mercury and never should be eaten, while mahimahi can be eaten once a week. For a complete list of how often you can eat a variety of fish, go to www.oceansalive.org.

Digestive Enzymes

According to Jordan Rubin, raw foods such as fruits, vegetables, and blanched nuts provide our bodies with important enzymes to digest foods and all their powerful nutrients. However, when we eat cooked or processed foods, our pancreas must produce the enzymes needed to digest them. Without those enzymes, you are more prone to gas, bloating, heartburn, and other digestive issues. If you eat almost all your food cooked or from bags, cans, and packages, chances are you have tired out your pancreas and consistently run low on enzymes. You can find a variety of enzymes at your local health food store. Rubin recommends Probio-Enzyme by GDRx and Omega Zyme by Garden of Life to name two.

DAILY JOURNAL & LOG

My unhealthy habit(s) is diminishing and my new habits are increasing in the following ways:

Nutrition and Fat Management

I ate for maximum energy and health today in the following ways:

- ☐ By drinking 4 to 6 ounces of water most waking hours.
- ☐ By eating protein and/or fiber at breakfast.
- ☐ By eating 3 to 4 vegetables.
- ☐ By eating 2 to 3 servings of fruits, whole grains, or nuts.

☐ By eating 5 to 6 snacks or small meals.

☐ By eating less from bags and boxes.

☐ By eating only when I was hungry.

☐ By eating 20 to 50 percent less food than usual in the last 4 hours of the day.

☐ By eating no more than 10 percent "empty" calories.

Rest and Regeneration

Last night I slept ___________ hours.

The quality of my sleep was: ________________

Tonight I will ____________________________ to ensure I get quality rest.

Today I managed my stress by:

Tomorrow I will unwind and relax by:

☐ I practiced deep breathing today for relaxation and health.

Fitness

☐ Today I did my minimum 10 minutes of exercise.

I exceeded the minimum by ____________________

Tomorrow I will improve or maintain my fitness by:

Thoughts for Today

day 15

Nourish Your Spirit—Testing for Truth

> For the time will come when they will not endure sound doctrine; but wanting to have their ears tickled, they will accumulate for themselves teachers in accordance with their own desires, and will turn away their ears from the truth and will turn aside to myths.
>
> 2 Timothy 4:3 NASB

Lose ten pounds in ten days! Look years younger in minutes!

Most of us are tired of these kinds of exaggerated claims. Yet sometimes we are still tempted by offers that speak to our weaknesses and promise results. It's been said that if it sounds too good to be true . . . it is. Fortunately, the single most important claim ever made in the history of humankind is true:

> The wages of sin is death, but the gift of God is eternal life in Christ Jesus our Lord.
>
> Romans 6:23

How often has a free gift turned out to be almost worthless? Yet, God in his mercy and grace offers us eternal life by faith alone in Christ . . . freely. This is a gift of incomprehensible value. To be a true believer and have assurance of salvation, we must believe that Christ is the only way to receive forgiveness for our sins, to give us access to God, and to provide an eternity for us in heaven. That truth is the foundation of our faith. Yet somewhere between salvation and the journey of sanctification (perfection—never realized this side of heaven), most of us take a few rabbit trails and shortcuts in our spiritual journey. On occasion we may allow our ears to be "tickled" by teaching that speaks directly to our personal needs.

Sometimes the words sound good and we don't take the time to test them against Scripture. If we do that too often, we can actually start believing myths and may even become New Age in our philosophy without even knowing it.

Just as we need to read the fine print on product claims, we need to discern the accuracy of everything we read, watch, or hear before we apply it to our lives. I love what my pastor, Tim Scott, used to say every day as we ended our daily talk radio show: "All that I taught you today, I believe is in accordance with the Word of God. But it is your responsibility to test it against the Word for yourself."

Without truth, we process our life circumstances and decisions through an incorrect grid. We claim promises that may not be real and practice prayers or rituals that are not biblical. We go searching for God's wisdom and will in the wrong places and wonder why our faith is shaky and our foundation unstable. If we believe a lie, we will live a lie.

It doesn't matter how sincerely we love God and desire to know truth. We may be a Christian of high integrity and moral courage, sincere in all we do. Yet, without absolute truth we are sincerely wrong. Without truth we are destined for failure. However, integrity coupled with absolute truth results in powerful victory in the Christian life.

Prayer

Holy God, your Word alone is perfect truth. Please forgive me for the times I have looked to sources that don't use your Word as the foundation of their teaching. Help me, Father, to have a discerning mind that quickly recognizes lies, even those that are beautifully cloaked in what may at first glance appear to be truth. I hunger for your truth alone. Help me to be faithful to the study and meditation of your perfect precepts. In Jesus's name, amen.

FROM THE DEVOTION ABOVE I HAVE IDENTIFIED . . .

The lie I believe:

The truth I now receive:

☐ ☐ ☐ I practiced healthy self-talk today (one to three times).

My key personal statement is:

☐ ☐ ☐ I have repeated that message at least three times today.

☐ I have written my personal statement above on an index card or in a journal that I can continue to read if I need renewal in this area.

Nourish Your Body—Me? Diabetes?

When someone mentions the word *diabetes*, what thoughts come to your mind? Perhaps you think, *That will never happen to me. I will never need to completely avoid sugar or take daily insulin injections.* But sadly because of the obesity epidemic in this country, we could soon have a diabetes epidemic as well. In fact, type-2 diabetes, once only found in adults, is now showing up in children at an alarming rate. If you have been overweight for an extended period of time or hold a large amount of fat in your belly region, you are potentially at risk.

When I think of diabetes, I think of a worn-out pancreas and overloaded fat cells that just can't take on the workload of processing excess carbohydrates effectively anymore. I think of the potential for blindness, stroke, and the loss of a limb. I think of a life cut short, possibly by decades. And the saddest part of all, most people can prevent it.

All carbohydrates ultimately turn to sugar in the body. Sugar stimulates the release of insulin, which is necessary to transport it out of the bloodstream and into fat cells because your body must maintain a very delicate blood sugar balance. All excess carbohydrate or sugar is turned to fat. Once your fat cells reach their maximum capacity, they end up becoming resistant to insulin. This results in an abnormally high blood sugar level simply because your body has run out of places to put the excess. A dangerous cycle continues until symptoms of diabetes motivate you to seek medical attention.

To stop excess fat production and return to healthy blood sugar levels, you must drastically reduce your intake of simple carbohydrates. This allows your body to rest and relearn how to utilize insulin more effectively.

Our bodies are fine-tuned machines that accommodate many abuses. But, when we indulge beyond our body's capacity to adapt, disease ensues. In diabetes, it is as if a night clerk at a hotel is knocking on every door to every room to see if the current guest can squeeze one more person into their room for the night. But, sadly every room is full, and the excess guests must wander in the halls, accumulate in the lobby, and diminish the quality of the hotel. If the clerk had just lit the No Vacancy sign outside and not allowed excess guests in, he would not have such a problem. Most people (whether at risk for diabetes or not) need to reduce their intake of refined carbohydrates, so they never run out of "room" for excess sugar when it is ingested on occasion.

DAILY JOURNAL & LOG

My unhealthy habit(s) is diminishing and my new habits are increasing in the following ways:

Nutrition and Fat Management

I ate for maximum energy and health today in the following ways:

- ☐ By drinking 4 to 6 ounces of water most waking hours.
- ☐ By eating protein and/or fiber at breakfast.
- ☐ By eating 3 to 4 vegetables.
- ☐ By eating 2 to 3 servings of fruits, whole grains, or nuts.
- ☐ By eating 5 to 6 snacks or small meals.
- ☐ By eating less from bags and boxes.
- ☐ By eating only when I was hungry.
- ☐ By eating 20 to 50 percent less food than usual in the last 4 hours of the day.
- ☐ By eating no more than 10 percent "empty" calories.

Rest and Regeneration

Last night I slept ____________ hours.

The quality of my sleep was: __________________

Tonight I will ______________________________ to ensure I get quality rest.

Today I managed my stress by:

Tomorrow I will unwind and relax by:

☐ I practiced deep breathing today for relaxation and health.

Fitness

☐ Today I did my minimum 10 minutes of exercise.

I exceeded the minimum by ______________________

Tomorrow I will improve or maintain my fitness by:

Thoughts for Today

day 16

Nourish Your Spirit—It's a Dog's Life

> But godliness with contentment is great gain. For we brought nothing into the world, and we can take nothing out of it. But if we have food and clothing, we will be content with that.
>
> 1 Timothy 6:6–8

Expectations and successes. Disappointments and failures. Sometimes it seems like we are on a never-ending roller coaster of experiences that set the tone for our lives. If we are reaching our goals and realizing success, we are happy. If we run into challenging circumstances or fail at something, we are sad. This is no way to live.

In my opinion, dogs "get" it. They understand what's important. I have a cute little beagle named Max that I bought while we lived in Europe. All the local Swiss Italians who saw him on the street with me would exclaim, "*Piccobello cannelino!*" which means "cute little dog." Max didn't care that he was cute or that people called him a funny name. He just liked the attention and the nice little pat he got from most strangers. In fact, Max is very content if we satisfy just a few basic needs. He loves to eat the same meal day after day. And if he gets some personal attention and a nice walk, his life is a total success. Oh . . . and lots of sleep. In fact, he's snoring right now at my feet as I write. *Molto stanco cannelino*—very tired little dog.

But in most people's eyes, Max doesn't compare with the newly famous beagle Uno, who is the first beagle ever to win best in show at the Westminster dog show in New York. Uno is the ultimate dog success. Quite frankly, Uno could care less about his newfound fame. Don't tell his owner and handler, but he doesn't even know he's a champ. He wants the same things Max does—a little love and a lot of food.

The apostle Paul tells the younger Timothy that living a godly life with contentment is great gain. He reminds him that he arrived with nothing and will leave the same way, and that he should be content with simply having his basic needs for food and clothing met. So, how are you doing in the contentment category lately? Like me, do you struggle with the difference between "needing" and "wanting"? If so, then perhaps like me you need a daily reality check to remind you of just how blessed you are even in the midst of sometimes difficult situations.

Paul writes in Philippians 4:11 that he learned the secret to being content. So, what is the secret? It is gratefulness for who God is and what he has already done. It is finding satisfaction in the basics, because God has already lavished us with forgiveness, eternal life, and a great reward in heaven. And, it is there, in heaven, that we will wear a crown as "best in show" because we are judged by the perfect life and sacrifice of Christ.

Prayer

Heavenly Father, thank you for loving me despite all my flaws. Forgive me for caring more what people think than what you think at times. Lord, I want to learn to be content no matter what circumstance I'm in, knowing that your love and forgiveness are the most important things I can ever receive. Please help me, Lord, to see my blessings accurately and to also interpret the trials of life accurately as well. I can do all things, as you give me strength. Amen.

FROM THE DEVOTION ABOVE I HAVE IDENTIFIED . . .

The lie I believe:

The truth I now receive:

☐ ☐ ☐ I practiced healthy self-talk today (one to three times).

My key personal statement is:

☐ ☐ ☐ I have repeated that message at least three times today.

☐ I have written my personal statement above on an index card or in a journal that I can continue to read if I need renewal in this area.

Nourish Your Body—More Reasons to Get Your Zzz's

There's no way around the fact that you must sleep. But trying to get by with the minimum amount is hurting you more than you may think. Getting enough zzz's is essential. Hopefully the following sleep facts will increase your motivation to hit the hay earlier.

Improve Your Memory

According to a Harvard study, people who were not allowed to sleep for thirty-five hours straight performed almost 20 percent worse on memory tests than people who got adequate sleep. It is thought that your brain actually does some filing of sorts during sleep to allow for storage of new information the next day. Your brain needs good quality and quantity of sleep to tune up its systems for maximum potential.

Improve Your Waistline

Two hormones that tell your body when to start and stop eating are greatly affected by lack of sleep. Sleep deprivation increases the "start" hormone, gherlin, and decreases the stop hormone, leptin. In addition, insufficient sleep also increases your cortisol levels, which also increase appetite. And to add insult to injury, too little sleep also slows your metabolism. Are you convinced to get your essential 7.5 to 8.5 hours per night yet? If not, read on!

Improve Your Face

Sleep deprivation impacts the ability of the body to get vital nutrients to your skin in sufficient amounts, resulting in sallow or washed-out looking skin, especially on the face. Our bodies use the first third of our sleep cycle to repair cells. If our sleep is consistently insufficient, that reparation time is limited. If we can see the results of too little sleep in our faces, just imagine what may be happening within our bodies!

Increase Your Life Span

Recent studies suggest that women who get less than seven hours of sleep per night may have mortality rates that are 21 percent higher than their well-rested counterparts. While the reasons are not yet well understood, lack of sleep has been associated with an increased incidence of high blood pressure, diabetes, and depression.

DAILY JOURNAL & LOG

My unhealthy habit(s) is diminishing and my new habits are increasing in the following ways:

Nutrition and Fat Management

I ate for maximum energy and health today in the following ways:

- ☐ By drinking 4 to 6 ounces of water most waking hours.
- ☐ By eating protein and/or fiber at breakfast.
- ☐ By eating 3 to 4 vegetables.
- ☐ By eating 2 to 3 servings of fruits, whole grains, or nuts.
- ☐ By eating 5 to 6 snacks or small meals.
- ☐ By eating less from bags and boxes.
- ☐ By eating only when I was hungry.
- ☐ By eating 20 to 50 percent less food than usual in the last 4 hours of the day.
- ☐ By eating no more than 10 percent "empty" calories.

Rest and Regeneration

Last night I slept ____________ hours.

The quality of my sleep was: ________________

Tonight I will ______________________________ to ensure I get quality rest.

Today I managed my stress by:

Tomorrow I will unwind and relax by:

☐ I practiced deep breathing today for relaxation and health.

Fitness

☐ Today I did my minimum 10 minutes of exercise.

I exceeded the minimum by ____________________

Tomorrow I will improve or maintain my fitness by:

Thoughts for Today

day 17

Nourish Your Spirit—Seize the Day

> This is the day the LORD has made; let us rejoice and be glad in it.
>
> Psalm 118:24

Consider your last twenty-four hours. On a scale from one to ten, how would you rate the past day? Go ahead—take a moment to give it a grade. Your answer may tell you more than you might think. In order to fully embrace life with total enthusiasm and joy, we need to "seize the day." The true meaning of the Latin term "carpe diem" means to make the most of the moment. It also implies to some that you are to "do what you feel" without regard for the consequences. I would encourage you to seize each day, each and every moment, *with* regard for the consequences. That is, make the most of celebrating life and honoring God with your attitude and actions.

Life is rich, complex, and mysterious. Look up from your to-do lists, frustrations, and challenges to rejoice about something in this very moment. Develop a mental focus that cultivates a heart of gratitude and thankfulness. Join with the psalmist in exclaiming, "This is the day the Lord has made; let us rejoice and be glad in it." Notice, he didn't place any qualifications for rejoicing—*if* your kids are respectful . . . *if* your boss appreciates your hard work . . . *if* your husband gives you the attention you desire. Yet when we have an attitude of joy, our influence on those in our lives is profound.

Seizing the day with an "abundance mentality" is about seeing that God is in control despite our circumstances. It is about knowing that his love for us is unconditional and perfect when we place our trust in him through faith in Christ. Letting go of expectations and celebrating that which is often taken for granted is a big part of seizing the day. Expectations dictate the way we think God's goodness should come to us—what kind of box life is supposed to come in. Why not seize the day as God has given it, with its challenges and joys . . . right now.

Mother Teresa said, "Yesterday is gone. Tomorrow has not yet come. We have only today. Let us begin."[1] While planning is important, we can miss the moment when more thought is given to the future than action is taken in the now. Now is where we live. Now is the place we experience God. Perhaps one day in heaven, time won't have the limits it has for us in this earthly life. But for now . . . now is where we live.

Prayer

Heavenly Father, thank you for this day. No matter what it holds for me, thank you that you have given me one more day of life. I choose to be glad and rejoice because you are in control and you love me. I realize that it is my responsibility to choose joy . . . and I do! In Jesus's name I pray, amen.

FROM THE DEVOTION ABOVE I HAVE IDENTIFIED . . .

The lie I believe:

The truth I now receive:

☐ ☐ ☐ I practiced healthy self-talk today (one to three times).

My key personal statement is:

☐ ☐ ☐ I have repeated that message at least three times today.

☐ I have written my personal statement above on an index card or in a journal that I can continue to read if I need renewal in this area.

Nourish Your Body—Acid-Alkaline Balance

Lack of energy, easily fatigued, inability to cope, frequently chilled, increased infections, high irritability, headaches, conjunctivitis, stomach problems and hyperacidity, diarrhea, abdominal cramps, kidney stones, respiratory complaints, dry skin, thin nails, leg cramps, and more could mean your body is too acidic. And chances are, unless you eat like a monkey, you are.

According to naturopathic doctor and author Christopher Vasey, despite the diversity of substances our body uses to build and function (to include amino acids, sugars, fatty acids, vitamins, minerals, and more), it is possible to classify them all into two major groups: alkaline

> or acid. These two different groups have opposing but complementary characteristics. To be healthy, the body needs both. When alkaline and acids are present in equal quantities, balance is achieved.[1]

The problem is that in our modern world, people eat more acidic foods than alkaline. In a nutshell, most vegetables, many fruits, and a few nuts are alkaline. The rest of what we eat (in general) is acidic. And the foods that hit the "extreme acid" list include our favorites: sugar, caffeine, most carbohydrates, soft drinks, alcohol, most grains, meat, poultry, and most packaged foods. No wonder we are super-acidic!

When we are young (under thirty-five), our bodies have better buffering systems to deal with our lopsided diets. But as we age, we lose that ability, and it becomes more and more critical to find balance.

In the past five or six years, I've started to have some issues related to my spine, specifically bone spurs and narrowing that are common as we age. After years of physical activity, I have learned how to exercise and maintain core strength so I can stay active for life. But I was really concerned when I noticed a spur on my shoulder just popping out like a little anthill and then a few months later a significant bump on my clavicle bone. Of course I saw my medical doctor, who confirmed it was a bone spur. He told me if it bothered me cosmetically, the only thing I could do is have it surgically removed. No thank you.

I got to thinking, *If I'm growing little "horns" on the outside of my body, what in the world is going on inside?* So I consulted my favorite naturopath (and old radio host buddy), Dr. Mark Stengler, and got some good advice. First, he told me that I was probably pulling excessive amounts of calcium from my bones (not a good thing for a menopausal woman) to neutralize my acidic body. Then when my body was done with the calcium, it was putting it back in strange places. The immediate need was to (1) take sufficient amounts of calcium, magnesium, and vitamin D (which I should have been taking anyway—once again . . . I'm still learning also); and (2) get my body much more alkaline to restore balance. I did just that, and with an added homeopathic dose of Calcarea fluorica, the bone spurs on my shoulder and clavicle look and feel smaller. I'm told not all bodies will reverse the process easily. And quite honestly, that is not the greatest benefit. When I keep my diet balanced, I have higher energy and brighter skin, and I sleep better. Not to mention I lost a little weight without even trying.

There are so many good reasons to bring our bodies into alkaline/acid balance. When they are out of balance, inflammation occurs all over the body. The easiest way to promote balance is to simply eat less of the foods we don't need anyway and then eat the acid foods we do need like proteins and complex carbohydrates in equal proportion to fruits, vegetables, and a few nuts. It is so much better to do the right things before you notice symptoms. I'm a very high energy woman. But this was one area of my life that was really out of whack.

You can measure your body's acid/alkaline balance by measuring the pH of your urine with test strips for that purpose. They are very inexpensive and available at most pharmacies. It is ideal to have a pH of about 7.0 in the middle of your day. Anything under that means your body is acid. You can learn much more about this important aspect of your health in a multitude of health books if you are interested. I hope that sharing this information will encourage you to be more mindful that your body may be working overtime when you continue to eat "out of balance."

DAILY JOURNAL & LOG

My unhealthy habit(s) is diminishing and my new habits are increasing in the following ways:

Nutrition and Fat Management

I ate for maximum energy and health today in the following ways:

- ☐ By drinking 4 to 6 ounces of water most waking hours.
- ☐ By eating protein and/or fiber at breakfast.
- ☐ By eating 3 to 4 vegetables.
- ☐ By eating 2 to 3 servings of fruits, whole grains, or nuts.
- ☐ By eating 5 to 6 snacks or small meals.
- ☐ By eating less from bags and boxes.
- ☐ By eating only when I was hungry.
- ☐ By eating 20 to 50 percent less food than usual in the last 4 hours of the day.
- ☐ By eating no more than 10 percent "empty" calories.

Rest and Regeneration

Last night I slept ____________ hours.

The quality of my sleep was: ________________

Tonight I will ______________________________ to ensure I get quality rest.

Today I managed my stress by:

Tomorrow I will unwind and relax by:

☐ I practiced deep breathing today for relaxation and health.

Fitness

☐ Today I did my minimum 10 minutes of exercise.

I exceeded the minimum by ____________________

Tomorrow I will improve or maintain my fitness by:

Thoughts for Today

day 18

Nourish Your Spirit—The Words of My Mouth

> But the things that come out of the mouth come from the heart, and these make a man "unclean."
>
> Matthew 15:18

The mouth can cause us so much trouble. From putting too much food in to letting the wrong words out, it is often a key player in many of our challenges. Too often, we say something before we've passed our thoughts through the filter of God's truth. Words that tear down and wound don't please God. Words that gossip or slander don't either. Yet it is so easy to want to share a juicy tidbit about someone or pass on some interesting news in the cloak of a "prayer request." I wonder how many of these kinds of prayer requests were ever really prayed about.

It seems if we can get to the root of controlling our mouth and our tongue, which we are told in James 3:6 "corrupts the whole person," we may be able to control our entire self. Our verse above says that what comes out of our mouths actually originates in our hearts. If we want to know the state of our own hearts, perhaps we should listen more carefully to not only the words we are speaking but also the silent conversations we are having inside our own minds. In the

Bible, the word *heart* refers to the soul. And the mind is the soul's pilot. As we have already learned, our words are by-products of our thoughts, and our thoughts originate from our beliefs. If we want our hearts to be pure and have words that flow naturally from our mouths, we must change our thinking.

If the words we are speaking are tearing down more than building up, we definitely need some "heart surgery," which begins by identifying the lies we believe so they can be excised from our minds. These are the "unclean" things that Matthew is speaking about.

Angry words come out of an angry heart and despairing words out of a desperate heart. Whatever negative, destructive words seem to flow out of our mouths freely and regularly reveal the condition of our hearts. But the opposite is true as well. Kind words flow from a kind heart, lovely words from a loving heart. By identifying our negative emotions and words, we can begin the process of transformation as we replace that which tears down with that which builds up.

As with all spiritual concerns, this is not a matter of self-control but rather of surrender and transformation. It took time for those lies to become imbedded, and it will take some time to dislodge them. As our hearts and minds become purified, so do our thoughts and our words. And surprisingly, a changed heart may also produce changed appetites for food and other things, as the "mouth" may no longer need to try to fill the gaps of a damaged heart.

Prayer

Holy God, forgive me for the words I speak at times that dishonor you and reveal the areas of my heart that need transformation. Please help me to become more aware of the words I speak and the condition of my heart. Help me identify the lies I believe and replace them with your transforming truth. I pray this in Jesus's precious name, amen.

FROM THE DEVOTION ABOVE I HAVE IDENTIFIED . . .

The lie I believe:

The truth I now receive:

☐ ☐ ☐ I practiced healthy self-talk today (one to three times).

My key personal statement is:

☐ ☐ ☐ I have repeated that message at least three times today.

☐ I have written my personal statement above on an index card or in a journal that I can continue to read if I need renewal in this area.

Nourish Your Body—Nix the Artificial

These days our bodies are bombarded with so many hidden chemicals. When we eat packaged food, chances are we'll get a hefty dose of preservatives. Even the lean meats and poultry we select are often laced with hormones and antibiotics. And, most frustrating of all, when we finally are convinced it's time to eat more fruits and veggies, we have to deal with pesticides.

So what's the solution? First, we really need to decrease our consumption of processed foods. Second, there are many markets all over the United States that offer hormone- and antibiotic-free meat and poultry. And third, some fruits and veggies can be washed to remove many of the pesticides. It is advisable whenever possible (and the food budget permits) to go organic when it comes to things like berries, broccoli, and other produce that is harder to scrub clean. Obviously fruits that need to be peeled are no issue. And by the way, most nutritionists still recommend eating lots and lots of fruits and veggies even if they are not organic. The benefits will always outweigh the downside.

But there is a set of chemicals that many dieters purposely ingest and put into their foods every day—artificial sweeteners. As I've already discussed, no matter the brand, they all have a significant downside in the body as these once "natural substances," now altered in the laboratory, enter your body. Not only do you risk your health by continuing to use these products—you actually risk gaining weight!

According to an article written by leading health expert Dr. Joseph Mercola:

> Foods and beverages that contain no-calorie artificial sweeteners may be ruining your ability to control your food intake and body weight, according to new research by psychologists at Purdue University's Ingestive Behavior Research Center. In their study, when compared with rats that ate yogurt sweetened with glucose (a simple sugar), rats that ate yogurt sweetened with the zero-calorie artificial sweetener saccharin:
>
> Consumed more calories (and didn't make up for it by cutting back later). They gained more weight and put on more body fat.
>
> It's thought that consuming artificial sweeteners breaks the connection between a sweet sensation and a high-calorie food, thereby changing your body's ability to regulate intake. The researchers also measured the rats' core body temperatures, which typically rise after eating. However, after eating a sweet, high-calorie meal, rats that ate saccharin had a lower rise in body temperature than rats that ate glucose. The researchers believe that this blunted biological response led the rats to overeat, and made it harder to burn off the calories later.[1]

DAILY JOURNAL & LOG

My unhealthy habit(s) is diminishing and my new habits are increasing in the following ways:

Nutrition and Fat Management

I ate for maximum energy and health today in the following ways:

- ☐ By drinking 4 to 6 ounces of water most waking hours.
- ☐ By eating protein and/or fiber at breakfast.
- ☐ By eating 3 to 4 vegetables.
- ☐ By eating 2 to 3 servings of fruits, whole grains, or nuts.
- ☐ By eating 5 to 6 snacks or small meals.
- ☐ By eating less from bags and boxes.
- ☐ By eating only when I was hungry.
- ☐ By eating 20 to 50 percent less food than usual in the last 4 hours of the day.
- ☐ By eating no more than 10 percent "empty" calories.

Rest and Regeneration

Last night I slept ____________ hours.

The quality of my sleep was: ________________

Tonight I will ______________________________ to ensure I get quality rest.

Today I managed my stress by:

Tomorrow I will unwind and relax by:

☐ I practiced deep breathing today for relaxation and health.

Fitness

☐ Today I did my minimum 10 minutes of exercise.

I exceeded the minimum by ____________________

Tomorrow I will improve or maintain my fitness by:

Thoughts for Today

day 19

Nourish Your Spirit—Prayer Protection

> When he rose from prayer and went back to the disciples, he found them asleep, exhausted from sorrow. "Why are you sleeping?" he asked them. "Get up and pray so that you will not fall into temptation."
>
> Luke 22:45–46

Have you noticed how much more emotional and weak you feel when you are sad, hungry, or tired? Some people get grouchy, others act downright angry, and some run to the cover of sleep. But everyone has less tenacity and resolve to make the right choices and do the right things when they are in such a state. It seems like a switch in our brains flips off and we are no longer our old selves. So what are we to do when we are in this weakened state? It seems from the passage above, and others, that the wisest and most beneficial thing to do is pray.

Jesus needed his disciples more than ever that last night in the garden as he poured out his heart to God and prepared to die. Yet, of all times, they failed him because they were exhausted. He knew they were vulnerable, and so he gave them the best advice possible: "Get up and pray so that you will not fall into temptation." When our minds and hearts get stuck on the thing that is taking us down into frustration or despair, it is best to change our focus and look up to God in prayer. Prayer is always the right thing to do, whether our crisis is life-and-death or simply one more nagging little temptation that usually wins the war of our will.

What should you do when the junk food is calling your name, the mall is drawing you in with all the fabulous sales, or your desire to be a couch potato is overriding your desire to have a healthy body? Pray. Prayer immediately acknowledges you are in a battle, and you need to submit your will to God rather than your own weak flesh. It may seem silly to pray to avoid the Oreos, but Paul told us in 1 Thessalonians 5:17 to "pray continually" and in Philippians 4:6 that "in everything, by prayer and petition, with thanksgiving, present your requests to God." Everything includes your battle with Oreos. When we are "looking up," our focus is on God. When we are "looking in," our focus is on ourselves and our immediate gratification. When you are facing temptation on any level . . . get up and pray!

Prayer

Heavenly Father, thank you for the power of prayer and that it changes me and protects me from temptation. Please help me to remember to pray at the first moment of temptation and to surrender my immediate gratification and rather be focused on your glorification. I pray this in the mighty name of Jesus. Amen.

FROM THE DEVOTION ABOVE I HAVE IDENTIFIED . . .

The lie I believe:

The truth I now receive:

☐ ☐ ☐ I practiced healthy self-talk today (one to three times).

My key personal statement is:

☐ ☐ ☐ I have repeated that message at least three times today.

☐ I have written my personal statement above on an index card or in a journal that I can continue to read if I need renewal in this area.

Nourish Your Body—Active Lifestyle Choices

As you have already learned, small steps taken consistently can add up in a big way over time in all areas of your life. To follow are some simple ideas that you can incorporate into every day to increase your energy, improve your fitness, and burn more calories.

Idea #1: Once a day, take about five seconds to jump up and down to stimulate your bones and increase your circulation. Make sure you are wearing supportive shoes and are not on a concrete surface. Do this every day and your bones will be stronger. Warning: only do this if you do not have back or other structural issues.

Idea #2: Take five- to ten-minute exercise breaks whenever you can. If the idea of getting up an hour early to get in a complete workout doesn't "work out" for you, just do what you can in small increments. It *will* add up. March in place while you watch the morning news before you jump in the shower. Take a short walk after lunch before returning to your usual routine. When you go shopping, park at the farthest corner of the parking lot. After dinner, do your sit-ups and other conditioning exercises while you chat with family, watch a favorite show, or listen to energizing music.

Idea #3: Make it a new habit to take two to three minutes every two hours to incorporate some basic stretches into your daily routine. If you sit at a desk, stand up and roll your shoulders back ten to twelve times followed by a quad stretch for the front of your thighs by grabbing your foot with one hand and pulling your heel toward your buttocks. If you spend a lot of time on your feet, stretch your calves by standing on a step and dropping your heel lower than the step on one side and then the other. When you are exhausted from a long day, lie on the floor and do a variety of stretches while you watch TV or simply enjoy some quietness.

Idea #4: Never stand when you can pace; never ride when you can walk. When you are waiting for someone or something, pace or walk short distances to pass the time. Take the stairs whenever you can. Whenever I'm in airports and must make a connecting flight, I rarely take the underground trains but rather walk the entire distance to my gate—sometimes up to a mile! And when I'm standing at the back of the plane, waiting to use the restroom, I always do stretches.

You can find creative ways to improve your fitness even on busy days if you try. Those little things can prevent overuse injuries, increase your sense of well-being, and enhance your health. Try it!

DAILY JOURNAL & LOG

My unhealthy habit(s) is diminishing and my new habits are increasing in the following ways:

Nutrition and Fat Management

I ate for maximum energy and health today in the following ways:

- ☐ By drinking 4 to 6 ounces of water most waking hours.
- ☐ By eating protein and/or fiber at breakfast.
- ☐ By eating 3 to 4 vegetables.
- ☐ By eating 2 to 3 servings of fruits, whole grains, or nuts.
- ☐ By eating 5 to 6 snacks or small meals.
- ☐ By eating less from bags and boxes.
- ☐ By eating only when I was hungry.
- ☐ By eating 20 to 50 percent less food than usual in the last 4 hours of the day.
- ☐ By eating no more than 10 percent "empty" calories.

Rest and Regeneration

Last night I slept ____________ hours.

The quality of my sleep was: _________________

Tonight I will ______________________________ to ensure I get quality rest.

Today I managed my stress by:

Tomorrow I will unwind and relax by:

☐ I practiced deep breathing today for relaxation and health.

Fitness

☐ Today I did my minimum 10 minutes of exercise.

I exceeded the minimum by ____________________

Tomorrow I will improve or maintain my fitness by:

Thoughts for Today

day 20

Nourish Your Spirit—Walking on Water

> Then Peter got down out of the boat, walked on the water and came toward Jesus. But when he saw the wind, he was afraid and, beginning to sink, cried out, "Lord, save me!"
>
> Immediately Jesus reached out his hand and caught him. "You of little faith," he said, "why did you doubt?"
>
> Matthew 14:29–31

The closest that I've ever come to walking on water is waterskiing. And while that takes little or no faith, it does take focus. From the moment I yell "Hit it!" to the driver of the boat, I must put my full attention toward the feel of the rope, the ski, and my balance as I quickly come out of the water and glide on its surface. If I get distracted even for a split second, I'm going down.

Sometimes in our walk of faith, we are so captivated by the power and majesty of God that we can sense his presence and power in our lives in profound ways. But if we take our focus off of him and turn it instead to our own ability, we often lose confidence and find ourselves falling into old patterns of fear, frustration, and failure.

In the passage above, I can just see Peter—so excited to see the Lord that he jumps out of the boat before even considering his inability to walk on water. But Jesus rewards his faith with supernatural power *until* Peter changes his focus to the wind. I am also relieved that Jesus did not let him sink into the dark water before pulling him out, but rather he reached for him immediately. At first, when I read Jesus's words, "You of little faith," it sounded like a demoralizing criticism. But, then I realized when he asked, "Why did you doubt?" he is reminding Peter that his supernatural ability to walk on water came only because of his faith.

The Lord wants us to have strong faith to face the storms of life. When our faith falters, we falter. When our hope in Christ sinks, we sink. When the storm clouds of doubt come our way, we must look up to heaven and pray for the ability to see life's challenges through spiritual eyes. We must process every circumstance through the grid of God's Word. Only then will we have "walking on water" faith.

Prayer

Heavenly Father, all things are under your power. Please help me to see that nothing happens without your total awareness. Thank you for rescuing me again and again when I call out to you. Help me to grow in my faith and trust in you even when the storms of life make me feel insecure. In the mighty name of Jesus I pray. Amen.

FROM THE DEVOTION ABOVE I HAVE IDENTIFIED . . .

The lie I believe:

The truth I now receive:

☐ ☐ ☐ I practiced healthy self-talk today (one to three times).

My key personal statement is:

☐ ☐ ☐ I have repeated that message at least three times today.

☐ I have written my personal statement above on an index card or in a journal that I can continue to read if I need renewal in this area.

Nourish Your Body—Water Above All

Water . . . pure, fresh water. Every cell in your body craves it. Every system of your body needs it to function optimally. You exercise better, burn fat more efficiently, and have more energy when you are well hydrated. We live in a land that has water in abundance. Since an adult body is 50 to 70 percent water, it makes sense to give this key nutrient that sustains our lives more attention. Without it, our body's survival time is limited to a matter of hours or days. So why are so many people subclinically dehydrated? Probably because we drink too many things that quench our thirst and satisfy our appetites, like soda and coffee, and not enough simple, pure water.

Just imagine that each cell in your body is like a grape. When you don't drink enough water, your cells begin to look like raisins. And, of course, your muscle tissue also needs to stay plump since it is about 75 percent water. Most importantly, your blood is about 90 percent water. When you don't drink enough, your blood actually becomes thicker and your body becomes less efficient at transporting nutrients to all the cells in your body and carrying waste products from the cells to the kidneys for excretion in urine.

Your body will always deal with the most important bodily functions first. It needs sufficient water to do its work, so you should drink at least eight to ten glasses a day and more on days you exercise, due to increased sweating and breathing. Here's why: the average person loses ten cups of water per day—two cups to sweating and evaporation, two cups to breathing, and six cups to waste removal. You can replace up to two cups through the water in the foods you eat, but you have to make up the remaining eight cups by drinking fluids, preferably pure water. Dehydration causes numerous symptoms including fatigue, poor concentration, headaches, blurred vision, and lack of neuromuscular control.

When you are hungry, start off with a glass of fresh water. If you are feeling low on energy or if something hurts (like a headache), drink a glass of water. If you wait to drink water until you are thirsty, you are already dehydrated. So drink at least four to eight ounces every hour you're awake, whether you feel like it or not. The best way to develop a water habit is to have it with you at all times—in your car, at your desk, at the bathroom sink when you're getting ready in the morning. Carry your water bottle with you everywhere and drink up!

DAILY JOURNAL & LOG

My unhealthy habit(s) is diminishing and my new habits are increasing in the following ways:

Nutrition and Fat Management

I ate for maximum energy and health today in the following ways:

- ☐ By drinking 4 to 6 ounces of water most waking hours.
- ☐ By eating protein and/or fiber at breakfast.
- ☐ By eating 3 to 4 vegetables.
- ☐ By eating 2 to 3 servings of fruits, whole grains, or nuts.
- ☐ By eating 5 to 6 snacks or small meals.
- ☐ By eating less from bags and boxes.
- ☐ By eating only when I was hungry.
- ☐ By eating 20 to 50 percent less food than usual in the last 4 hours of the day.
- ☐ By eating no more than 10 percent "empty" calories.

Rest and Regeneration

Last night I slept ____________ hours.

The quality of my sleep was: __________________

Tonight I will ________________________________ to ensure I get quality rest.

Today I managed my stress by:

Tomorrow I will unwind and relax by:

☐ I practiced deep breathing today for relaxation and health.

Fitness

☐ Today I did my minimum 10 minutes of exercise.

I exceeded the minimum by ______________________

Tomorrow I will improve or maintain my fitness by:

Thoughts for Today

day 21

Nourish Your Spirit—Choosing the Best from All the Good

> "Everything is permissible for me"—but not everything is beneficial. "Everything is permissible for me"—but I will not be mastered by anything. "Food for the stomach and the stomach for food"—but God will destroy them both.
>
> 1 Corinthians 6:12–13

"American Express . . . don't leave home without it," says the television commercial voice as images of attractive people dine, travel, and shop as if there is no tomorrow. I have an American Express card, and the company allows me to charge thousands and thousands of dollars on it whenever I want. It's permissible . . . but certainly not beneficial to my budget!

The voice coming from the McDonald's drive-through menu asks, "Would you like to supersize that?" It's your choice . . . it's permissible. If you drive through often (with or without supersizing), one thing is sure—*you* will be supersized. So many things in life are left up to our free will, even spiritual matters. Some things are not an issue of sin but rather an issue of value. When we let our human appetites get out of control, they can become our master with what seems like a power of their own.

As New Testament believers, we are no longer under the law. We live under the new covenant of grace. We no longer tithe under compulsion but out of love for God. We have so much freedom and liberty to worship God. And yet too often we worship those things that gratify our own cravings more than that which glorifies God.

Edwin Louis Cole once said, "Everything is under the power of choice. But once a choice is made, we become a servant to that choice."[1] When we make choices that are not well thought out, or practice behaviors that are taken to excess and become bad habits, what was once liberty soon becomes bondage.

The apostle Paul is a consistent role model of someone who is totally sold out to Christ on every level. As we read in the Scripture above, he knew he had great freedom, yet his first priority was to always choose the best (the beneficial) from all the good. He was wise enough to know the risk of becoming a slave to uncontrolled indulgence. As we make choices each day, here are a few questions we can ask ourselves that may help us determine how to choose the best from all the good:

Will it help me know and love God more?
Will it help me know and love my spouse more?
Will it help me know and love my children more?
Will it help me grow in loving others more?

Prayer

Dear Lord, please forgive me for the bad choices I have made in the past. Thank you for the liberty you give me. Help me to be wise enough to choose the best from all the good. Mold me into the person you desire me to be so that my desires are in sync with yours. Help me to delight in what delights you. May I be mastered only by you, Lord. Amen.

FROM THE DEVOTION ABOVE I HAVE IDENTIFIED . . .

The lie I believe:

The truth I now receive:

☐ ☐ ☐ I practiced healthy self-talk today (one to three times).

My key personal statement is:

☐ ☐ ☐ I have repeated that message at least three times today.

☐ I have written my personal statement above on an index card or in a journal that I can continue to read if I need renewal in this area.

Nourish Your Body—Excuses . . . Excuses

It's been said that all excuses are equal and are all equally worthless. Wow. That seems pretty harsh. But if you think about it, most excuses don't really help get you where you want to go . . . they just help you justify staying stuck. I've listed three of the most popular reasons why people don't stick to improved nutrition or fitness plans. Let's take each one and tear apart the excuse and replace it with a healthier action.

Excuse #1: I Can't Resist My Favorite Foods

Your favorite foods will always be available to you. Don't try to live by a nutrition plan that completely eliminates them. Then you will want them all the more. Tell yourself that you can have anything you want, whenever you want it, but you choose to have those foods only on occasion and in moderation because you want a lean, healthy body even more. Give yourself little goals for rewarding yourself with your favorite food. And when you do have it, tell yourself as you are eating it how quickly you are satisfied and how it is really not as wonderful as you once thought. You'll be amazed over time how your ability to resist grows.

Excuse #2: I Don't Have Enough Time

We all have the same twenty-four hours in every day, and we choose to make time for that which is most important to us. If you have not taken the time to exercise, shop for healthy food, or take any number of positive lifestyle steps, it wasn't important enough. Except for the rarest of occasions (when we are in crisis mode due to outside circumstances), most of us can find an extra thirty to sixty minutes in our day to invest in our lifestyle. Do you watch television or waste precious time looking at every single email you receive? It is amazing how much time could be redistributed to something more profitable. It may take a while to create enough balance in your life to allow some margin for your body. But if you never take it now, you will pay at some point. You pay now or you pay later . . . but you always pay.

Excuse #3: I Don't See Results Fast Enough

When we have an average headache and take a pain reliever, our headache is usually gone within half an hour. If our hairstyle is outdated, we go and get a new look and there's an instant change. But losing weight, increasing your energy, and getting fit are not "quick fixes." The first thing you have to do with this excuse is make yourself accept reality. The difference between reality and unrealistic expectations is called your "misery factor." The reality is that it will take time to notice significant change. Do it anyway. Measure your success by the changes you are making daily as you log your success.

DAILY JOURNAL & LOG

My unhealthy habit(s) is diminishing and my new habits are increasing in the following ways:

Nutrition and Fat Management

I ate for maximum energy and health today in the following ways:

- ☐ By drinking 4 to 6 ounces of water most waking hours.
- ☐ By eating protein and/or fiber at breakfast.
- ☐ By eating 3 to 4 vegetables.
- ☐ By eating 2 to 3 servings of fruits, whole grains, or nuts.
- ☐ By eating 5 to 6 snacks or small meals.
- ☐ By eating less from bags and boxes.
- ☐ By eating only when I was hungry.
- ☐ By eating 20 to 50 percent less food than usual in the last 4 hours of the day.
- ☐ By eating no more than 10 percent "empty" calories.

Rest and Regeneration

Last night I slept ____________ hours.

The quality of my sleep was: __________________

Tonight I will ________________________________ to ensure I get quality rest.

Today I managed my stress by:

Tomorrow I will unwind and relax by:

☐ I practiced deep breathing today for relaxation and health.

Fitness

☐ Today I did my minimum 10 minutes of exercise.

I exceeded the minimum by ____________________

Tomorrow I will improve or maintain my fitness by:

Thoughts for Today

day 22

Nourish Your Spirit—Joyful . . . Prayerful . . . Thankful

> Be joyful always; pray continually; give thanks in all circumstances, for this is God's will for you in Christ Jesus.
>
> 1 Thessalonians 5:16–18

The movie *Pollyanna* was one of my favorites when I was a child. The title character was an orphan girl who went to live with her sour aunt Polly after her parents died. Pollyanna continually played a little mind game her father had called the "glad game," where she always found a way to turn something negative into something positive. Often her attitude was uplifting and contagious; and other times it was downright unrealistic. As a result the term "Pollyanna" refers to a person who is regarded as being foolishly or blindly optimistic.

But perhaps we can learn something from Pollyanna about choosing joy as a response to difficult situations. If we are told in Scripture to be joyful, prayerful, and thankful in all circumstances, then it must be possible. But can we be all those things even at death's door?

When the evangelist D. L. Moody was dying, his son was at his bedside and heard him say in quiet words, "Earth recedes: heaven opens before me." His son thought that his father was dreaming and began to rouse him when the elder Moody exclaimed, "No, this is no dream, Will. It is beautiful! If this is death, it is sweet! God is calling me and I must go."[1]

Even in death, God's will for us is to be joyful, prayerful, and thankful. We need to practice seeing every single thing through spiritual eyes, trying to grasp the whole picture of God's plan despite our limited capacity to see it in its entirety. Life can be painful, even devastating at times. Yet we must remember that our pain is only temporary and our heavenly Father is always present, ready to hear every word uttered to him in prayer.

Life is much like a pregnant woman going through labor. The contractions represent the difficult, sometimes painful periods of life we all endure. The breaks between each labor pain are the times when life is peaceful or rewarding. The pregnant woman knows that the contractions are necessary to reach her goal of delivering her newborn child. And though in pain, she tries to keep her mind on the ultimate goal. Like that laboring mother, we must ride the contractions of life with our eye on our ultimate prize, which is perfection in heaven with Christ. If we learn how to keep our focal point always on the Lord, we can remain joyful, prayerful, and thankful throughout the labors of life.

Prayer

Dear heavenly Father, it is so hard to consistently live with a joyful, prayerful, and thankful attitude. Please help me to refocus my attention on the truth of who I am in you and the promises you have made me for now and eternity. Increase my faith and help me rest in your powerful truth so that I can live in daily joy and gratitude. In Jesus's name, amen.

FROM THE DEVOTION ABOVE I HAVE IDENTIFIED . . .

The lie I believe:

The truth I now receive:

☐ ☐ ☐ I practiced healthy self-talk today (one to three times).

My key personal statement is:

☐ ☐ ☐ I have repeated that message at least three times today.

☐ I have written my personal statement above on an index card or in a journal that I can continue to read if I need renewal in this area.

Nourish Your Body—Energy Crisis

My energy bill was outrageously high a few years ago. It seemed like no matter what I did, each month's charges grew. I think I could faintly hear the sound of coins clinking in my pipes as my energy budget went down the drain. Every light left on . . . clink. Every unattended television and radio left on . . . clink, clink. Every long, hot shower . . . clink, clink, clink. Little by little, I found creative, small steps to slow down the "clinking." It didn't seem to make a big difference at first. But our recent bill reflects considerable improvement.

If your body could use an "energy tune-up," small steps can add up in your physical dimension as well. To improve your health and vitality, try these simple lifestyle tips. Over time, your energy reserves will increase, and if you're consistent you might have energy to spare. Just remember, it takes more than three or four days for these small steps to add up. Do the best you can to start improving a little each day in the areas where you have the most trouble.

Step 1: Catch a Few More Zzz's

Sound obvious? It is. But many people who experience low energy don't get enough sleep. Deep, dreaming (REM) sleep is the time when your body undergoes cellular renewal. If you want to stay young longer and feel great, get enough sleep. For most people, it is simply an issue of planning, prioritizing, and winding down earlier.

Step 2: Guzzle More Pure, Fresh Water

The number one nutritional reason for low energy is subclinical dehydration. You can be a "quart low" and never feel thirsty. At the first sign of fatigue, drink a tall glass of water. Better yet, drink four to six ounces every hour you are awake and even more when you are exercising.

Step 3: Cut Back on Caffeine

Now, you're really in a panic. Caffeine may be your energy savior. But in reality, caffeine only gives you a short burst of energy. It gets your adrenaline pumping and heart rate racing, but once the initial buzz is gone, you'll end up more tired. And caffeine will rob you of water, the natural energizer. If you're a coffee lover like me, switch to quality decafs, and even limit those to no more than two cups per day. I've fooled a lot of people by serving them decaf without their knowledge. Try it . . . you'll like it.

Step 4: Rev Up Your Engine with Activity

You may be thinking, *If I'm already exhausted, more activity or exercise is going to deplete me even more.* The opposite is true. Purposeful aerobic activity like walking, swimming, and biking increases your circulation, stimulates your metabolism, and generates lots of feel-good hormones.

Step 5: Lose the Sugar Bowl

Like caffeine, sugar brings you up, up, up and then drops you like a hot potato. You don't have to be a purist and avoid sugar completely. If you can limit empty calories and sweets until well after lunch, your cravings will diminish and your energy will stay higher.

Step 6: Eat for High Energy

Build a nutritional foundation with adequate protein and high fiber. Your energy after lunch will be influenced by the quality of your breakfast, and your energy in the evening by the quality of your lunch. Both protein and fiber stabilize your blood sugar to keep your energy up and your hunger down. Doesn't it make sense that breakfast and lunch deserve the highest-quality foods? Most people eat their biggest portion of protein (and calories) at dinner when they need it least. Try beefing up your nutrition early in the day to improve your energy. Most people don't need a major meal at dinner. Why not eat more complete meals early in the day and enjoy a light snack or dessert instead of dinner?

Try one or more of these energizing tips over the next few weeks. You'll be amazed at how much better you can feel when you energize from the inside out!

DAILY JOURNAL & LOG

My unhealthy habit(s) is diminishing and my new habits are increasing in the following ways:

Nutrition and Fat Management

I ate for maximum energy and health today in the following ways:

- ☐ By drinking 4 to 6 ounces of water most waking hours.
- ☐ By eating protein and/or fiber at breakfast.
- ☐ By eating 3 to 4 vegetables.
- ☐ By eating 2 to 3 servings of fruits, whole grains, or nuts.
- ☐ By eating 5 to 6 snacks or small meals.
- ☐ By eating less from bags and boxes.
- ☐ By eating only when I was hungry.
- ☐ By eating 20 to 50 percent less food than usual in the last 4 hours of the day.
- ☐ By eating no more than 10 percent "empty" calories.

Rest and Regeneration

Last night I slept ____________ hours.

The quality of my sleep was: ________________

Tonight I will ______________________________ to ensure I get quality rest.

Today I managed my stress by:

Tomorrow I will unwind and relax by:

☐ I practiced deep breathing today for relaxation and health.

Fitness

☐ Today I did my minimum 10 minutes of exercise.

I exceeded the minimum by ____________________

Tomorrow I will improve or maintain my fitness by:

Thoughts for Today

day 23

Nourish Your Spirit—When You Fast

> When you fast, do not look somber as the hypocrites do, for they disfigure their faces to show men they are fasting. I tell you the truth, they have received their reward in full. But when you fast, put oil on your head and wash your face, so that it will not be obvious to men that you are fasting, but only to your Father, who is unseen; and your Father, who sees what is done in secret, will reward you.
>
> Matthew 6:16–18

Jesus did not say "*if* you fast," he said "*when* you fast." I guess that means he expects us to do just that . . . and all the while, keeping it just between God and us. So, if we are to fast, why? Is it for the reward spoken of in Matthew 6:18 above?

As a young Christian, I was afraid to fast because of my past eating disorder. As I've matured and found complete victory in that area of my life, occasional fasts have drawn me closer to God and given me clarity. One such fast was done before launching our Women of Purpose ministry in San Diego in 1997. Throughout the entire time, I sensed God's power and provision. The night we launched the ministry, over one hundred women attended from over twenty churches; and today, eleven years later, we have reached over three thousand women with the gospel. I know it was not the fast that gave our ministry its wings but rather God who heard our heart's cry for the lost and drew women to partner with us.

Fasting is spoken of in the Bible seventy-four times, and there are several recorded reasons why people fasted. These reasons include mourning someone's death, repentance and confession, seeking protection, seeking direction, healing from sickness, and sending people out for the purpose of ministry. As I prayed about today's devotion, I sensed God wants us to better understand this important element of the Christian walk—especially for those of us who have or still battle with eating issues. So this may seem a bit more instructional than inspirational today as we take a little extra time to seek clarity about how and when God calls us to fast. Since I am such a novice at fasting, I sought the wisdom of someone well grounded in this area. Dennis Rupert, pastor of New Life Community Church in Safford, Virginia, is that person; and by his permission, I am sharing his excellent teaching on this subject below—excerpted from the church website at www.new-life.net/fasting.htm, where you can read it in its entirety.

Thoughts on Fasting

The Bible tells us that food was given for four reasons: enjoyment, sustenance, fellowship, and worship. Yet, God also has a place for fasting in our lives. We must never think of fasting as a hunger strike designed to force God's hand and get our own way. We don't need to strong-arm God. God is good and eager to answer our prayers. He is generous and eager to give us good things. Don't use fasting to try to push God into a corner. Who knows? Maybe he would rather let you starve and join him in heaven!

What exactly does fasting (not eating food) mean? Why did people in the Bible "not eat"? We find a clue in Leviticus 16:29. This verse says that fasting is synonymous with "afflicting one's soul." We gain some insight here about how the Hebrews viewed fasting. Fasting is more than just "afflicting one's body." It is "afflicting one's soul." In other words, fasting in the Hebrew mind is something my soul participates in. Fasting is denying myself. It is denying not only my own body but also my own desires. It is a way of saying that food and my desires are secondary to something else. Fasting is an act of self-denial. But it is not only that and thus the reason God is not moved by religious hypocrisy.

Biblical fasting is "not eating" with spiritual communication in mind. We know this because it always occurs together with prayer in the Bible—ALWAYS. You can pray without fasting, but you cannot fast (biblically speaking) without praying. Biblical fasting is deliberately abstaining from food for a spiritual reason: *communication and relationship with the Father*. We also always find fasting connected with a very troubled spirit or anxious heart before the Lord. Fasting is something you do when you have a consuming reason to seek God for very special guidance, provision, or forgiveness. We fast to demonstrate that we are seeking God "with all our heart." Fasting puts things in proper focus. It is a physical way of saying,

"Food and the things of this life are not as important to me now as (fill in the blank)."

So when should a Christian fast? We should fast when we sense the Spirit of God leading us to do so. The occasion for fasting is a totally voluntary decision. A Christian may decide to fast whenever there is a spiritual concern or struggle in his or her life. Of course, there may be times when those in authority over us proclaim a fast, as was done by King Saul (1 Sam. 14:24) or Jehoshaphat (2 Chron. 20:3). But normally and ultimately that decision is solely between us and the Lord. It is important to understand that we cannot fast and pray expecting God to bless us when there is known sin in our lives. Fasting does not impress God with our spirituality to the point that he ignores our disobedience. On the contrary, genuine fasting will always cause us to examine our hearts to make sure everything is right with him.

In the Bible three basic fasts are recorded. The first, the "normal fast," was when a person abstained from food and liquid for a period of one day (from sunset to sunset). The second, the "partial fast," placed an emphasis on restriction of diet, rather than abstaining completely from eating, as in the prophet Daniel's fast recorded in Daniel 10:3. The last is the "radical fast," which is one in which the person refrains from both food and water or simply food for an extended period of time. A radical fast can be harmful to your health and in most cases should not exceed three days. Fasts that extend beyond three or seven days can be found in the Bible, but these exceptions were based upon direct guidance from God or a supernatural ability given by God to complete the fast. Examples of these extreme fasts are Moses (Deut. 9:9–18 and Exod. 34:28); Elijah (1 Kings 19:8); and Jesus (Matt. 4:1–11). We must be wise to fast based on our body's unique need or weakness. God is not so concerned with the "how" but rather the "heart."

God said, "When you seek me with all your heart, I will be found by you" (Jer. 29:13–14). When a man or woman is willing to set aside the legitimate appetites of the body to concentrate on the work of praying, they are demonstrating that they mean business and are seeking God with all their heart. Fasting is an expression of wholeheartedness.

Prayer

Dear God, please help me to know when you want me to fast and give me the strength to surrender my hunger and needs fully to you. I want to know you more intimately and understand how fasting fits into our relationship. I love you, Lord. Amen.

FROM THE DEVOTION ABOVE I HAVE IDENTIFIED . . .

The lie I believe:

The truth I now receive:

☐ ☐ ☐ I practiced healthy self-talk today (one to three times).

My key personal statement is:

☐ ☐ ☐ I have repeated that message at least three times today.

☐ I have written my personal statement above on an index card or in a journal that I can continue to read if I need renewal in this area.

Nourish Your Body—Fasting for Health

Fasting can serve two important purposes. First, as we already noted in our Nourish Your Spirit segment today, fasting is a way for believers to surrender themselves to the Lord and seek his forgiveness, wisdom, or provision during times of important decisions or trying circumstances.

The second reason to fast is for the health benefits it can provide. And while one may gain some health benefits from a spiritual fast, it is my personal opinion that this should not be the main motivation. Unfortunately for many who struggle with weight management issues or eating disorders, this may be a hard decision to make. I simply caution you to determine *which* objective you are seeking at the outset of your fast. God always deserves our best.

With that being said, let's take a quick look at some healthy ways to fast and their benefits. Regarding this subject, Jordan Rubin in his book *The Great Physician's Rx for Health and Wellness* writes, "I'm a firm believer in the value of giving the body's digestive system time off from the round-the-clock digestive cycle that so many people put their bodies under these days. Your liver—the hardest-working organ God gave you—will thank you."[1] He explains that to work efficiently, the liver needs the kind of rest that fasting or even healthy "undereating" on occasion provides.

Most people find that regular fasting (missing two to three simultaneous meals per week) helps them have higher energy, stay leaner, and promote a younger appearance. Jordan Rubin chooses to do a one-day partial fast almost every week by skipping breakfast and lunch and then eating a light dinner as a part of his total lifestyle plan.

If you have never fasted, you may want to start by simply eating only fruits and vegetables and drinking only water or herbal tea for two to three meals a week. As you begin to feel the benefits, you may want to try "water only" for a partial or whole day. Again, this type of fast is for the health benefits, so you can modify it in ways that maximize your ability to consider fasting as a regular part of your health regime.

As I stated elsewhere, the only proven way to increase longevity is to eat less, so fasting is certainly one way to do that. But, that being said, we also want to support a healthy metabolism. That requires that we eat at least as many calories as our RMR most of the time. Fasting for health purposes must maintain a balance between "resting and cleansing" your body with sustaining it. If you find yourself falling into an attitude of fasting for weight loss for days on end . . . *stop* fasting. We must maintain healthy and balanced attitudes about fasting (both spiritual and health related) in order to realize its benefits.

DAILY JOURNAL & LOG

My unhealthy habit(s) is diminishing and my new habits are increasing in the following ways:

Nutrition and Fat Management

I ate for maximum energy and health today in the following ways:

☐ By drinking 4 to 6 ounces of water most waking hours.

☐ By eating protein and/or fiber at breakfast.

☐ By eating 3 to 4 vegetables.

☐ By eating 2 to 3 servings of fruits, whole grains, or nuts.

☐ By eating 5 to 6 snacks or small meals.

☐ By eating less from bags and boxes.

☐ By eating only when I was hungry.

☐ By eating 20 to 50 percent less food than usual in the last 4 hours of the day.

☐ By eating no more than 10 percent "empty" calories.

Rest and Regeneration

Last night I slept ____________ hours.

The quality of my sleep was: _________________

Tonight I will ______________________________ to ensure I get quality rest.

Today I managed my stress by:

Tomorrow I will unwind and relax by:

☐ I practiced deep breathing today for relaxation and health.

Fitness

☐ Today I did my minimum 10 minutes of exercise.

I exceeded the minimum by _____________________

Tomorrow I will improve or maintain my fitness by:

Thoughts for Today

day 24

Nourish Your Spirit—Treasures of the Heart

> But store up for yourselves treasures in heaven, where moth and rust do not destroy, and where thieves do not break in and steal. For where your treasure is, there your heart will be also.
>
> Matthew 6:20–21

I heard a story about a Special Olympics event that took place in Seattle, Washington. All of the contestants were physically or mentally disabled. Nine assembled at the starting line for the one-hundred-yard dash, and at the sound of the gun, they all started out, perhaps not really "dashing" but with pure enthusiasm to finish the race and win. One boy immediately tripped on the asphalt, tumbled head over heels, and began to cry. The other eight heard the boy cry and slowed down to look back. Upon seeing the fallen boy, they all turned around and went back—every single one of them. One girl with Down's syndrome knelt down and kissed her scraped-up opponent and said, "This will make it better." Then, all nine linked arms and walked across the finish line together. Everyone in the entire stadium stood up and began cheering and did not stop for several minutes.

In the race of life, we often lose focus on what is truly important. In business, we strive to be the best and sometimes in the heat of competition don't see the faces of the people who seem to be in the way of accomplishing our goal.

Sadly, even in ministry there can be many conflicts and unhealthy competition as people try to promote their own ideas or position. When we put people above projects and fellowship above fame and fortune, we are truly storing up treasures in heaven. The truth is, we can't take our accomplishments or acquisitions with us to heaven. The only thing that will meet us there are our brothers and sisters in Christ.

Some of those could be people who came to know him because you responded differently to them in the course of life. Perhaps you were like the handicapped children, who turned around in the midst of their race and helped the weakest one make his way across the finish line.

Prayer

Father God, help me to realize when I am giving more attention to storing up treasures here on earth instead of in heaven. Forgive me that I sometimes put my agenda ahead of people. Open my heart and mind to your divine appointments each day, that I may store up treasures of love in heaven, where neither rust nor moth will destroy. I ask these things in the powerful name of Jesus. Amen.

FROM THE DEVOTION ABOVE I HAVE IDENTIFIED . . .

The lie I believe:

The truth I now receive:

☐ ☐ ☐ I practiced healthy self-talk today (one to three times).

My key personal statement is:

☐ ☐ ☐ I have repeated that message at least three times today.

☐ I have written my personal statement above on an index card or in a journal that I can continue to read if I need renewal in this area.

Nourish Your Body—Stress Kills

God designed us with a mind that needs downtime, a soul that needs refreshment, and a body that needs sufficient, quality sleep within every twenty-four-hour cycle. Why do we often fight God's design and think it is noble to work like crazy and run at a frantic pace? It's been said that stress kills. While a certain amount of stress is healthy and moves us forward, too much persistent stress does "kill" us both physically and psychologically.

In her book *Simplify Your Time*, Marcia Ramsland states:

> Studies have shown we have more than two hundred inputs a day—email, mail, thoughts, decisions, memos, phone calls, and on and on the list goes. But our short-term memory only holds seven items at a time. This explains why we often feel overloaded.[1]

I learned many years ago that God doesn't give us more than we can handle. But we sure can give ourselves too much! And when we do . . . there is a price to pay. Edwin Louis Cole says that everything is under the power of choice. But once a choice is made, we become a servant to that choice. Sometimes, it takes a lot of work and "undoing" to make up for a poor decision. Here are a few more facts I've learned:

Overloaded people fail . . . like an airplane, we can only hold so much luggage!

When we take on too much . . . we don't really do well at anything.

To maximize your life . . . you'll have to minimize your load.

Our busy, stressed-out lifestyles are not normal, and we need to learn what a normal, balanced lifestyle really looks like. Dr. Richard Swenson calls it "margin" in his book of the same name. Restoring physical margin requires that we take personal responsibility for our health. One of the ways that I have restored margin into my life is to reduce my daily to-do list to the five most important things, knowing that if I have more than five, I rarely have time to complete everything on my list. Learning how to let go has been my greatest de-stressor. I also often ask myself the following two questions:

What is the worst thing that will happen if I don't get this thing done?
What difference will it make a week or a month from now?

The answer to those questions helps me put my need to achieve and complete in perspective. If I don't put things in perspective, I am likely to miss many of God's divine appointments with the people he puts in my life.

There are all kinds of techniques for dealing with stress, but the most important is to reinterpret your priorities. My pastor says the difference between reality and our expectations is our "misery factor." To lower your misery, lower your unrealistic expectations. In the process you will rediscover the joy of life.

DAILY JOURNAL & LOG

My unhealthy habit(s) is diminishing and my new habits are increasing in the following ways:

Nutrition and Fat Management

I ate for maximum energy and health today in the following ways:

- ☐ By drinking 4 to 6 ounces of water most waking hours.
- ☐ By eating protein and/or fiber at breakfast.
- ☐ By eating 3 to 4 vegetables.
- ☐ By eating 2 to 3 servings of fruits, whole grains, or nuts.

☐ By eating 5 to 6 snacks or small meals.

☐ By eating less from bags and boxes.

☐ By eating only when I was hungry.

☐ By eating 20 to 50 percent less food than usual in the last 4 hours of the day.

☐ By eating no more than 10 percent "empty" calories.

Rest and Regeneration

Last night I slept ____________ hours.

The quality of my sleep was: _________________

Tonight I will _______________________________ to ensure I get quality rest.

Today I managed my stress by:

Tomorrow I will unwind and relax by:

☐ I practiced deep breathing today for relaxation and health.

Fitness

☐ Today I did my minimum 10 minutes of exercise.

I exceeded the minimum by ______________________

Tomorrow I will improve or maintain my fitness by:

Thoughts for Today

day 25

Nourish Your Spirit—Waves of Deceit

> Then we will no longer be infants, tossed back and forth by the waves, and blown here and there by every wind of teaching and by the cunning and craftiness of men in their deceitful scheming. Instead, speaking the truth in love, we will in all things grow up into him who is the Head, that is, Christ.
>
> Ephesians 4:14–15

As a young girl, I grew up very near the ocean in Southern California. I loved to play in the waves and body surf. I had absolutely no fear. When I was about twelve, I was caught in a riptide. As I struggled to swim toward shore, the power of the ocean kept pulling me farther out. No matter how hard I swam, I made no progress. I was confused because I didn't know about riptides. If I had, I would have known that I needed to swim parallel to the shore until I passed through it and then swim toward shore. Fortunately, I remained calm (and perhaps even had supernatural intervention), because within minutes I was moving forward and quickly reached the shore, relieved to have my feet once again on solid ground.

It is essential as Christians for us to be wise to the waves of deceptive teaching that can catch us up like a riptide. Just loving God is not enough. We must know his Word and be able to discern truth from lies. My close friend who loves the Lord dearly got caught up in such a lie. She had been watching Oprah and became intrigued by a guest who was sharing all sorts of positive teaching about how we can achieve our dreams and fulfill all of our goals. She was so inspired by this woman that she went to her website and got DVDs of her teaching for many of her friends. When she handed the DVD to me and told me about it, I was immediately concerned. After I watched it, I was deeply troubled that she could not see the deception. I knew that she needed to be set straight and yet I did not want her to feel ashamed, so I prayed that God would help me to speak the truth in love.

When I saw her next, I said a quick prayer and brought up the subject she had so enthusiastically shared earlier. But before I could even speak, she shared that she had seen her pastor earlier that day and he told her he was writing a book exposing "The Secret" (the teaching she had seen on Oprah) for the lie that is was. She had responded with surprise followed by great concern for her own naivety. She proceeded to call all the friends to whom she had given the DVDs. God had answered my prayer beyond what I could have asked or imagined, and my dear friend had learned a valuable lesson.

Sadly, *The Secret* became a bestseller because it claims that the "universe" is obliged to deliver us anything that we consistently think about with focus and intent. Who wouldn't want this lie to be true? But, in truth, it pushes people further and further from the truth . . . and from the true and living God. As Christians, we must not only know truth by studying God's Word, we must also be ready to boldly "speak the truth in love" to our brothers and sisters in Christ when they get caught in a riptide of deception.

Prayer

Father God, thank you for your powerful, life-changing truth. Please help me to understand your Word and rely on it alone as my foundation for living. Help me to be discerning about false teaching and to boldly speak the truth in love when I need to help a brother or sister in Christ. Amen.

FROM THE DEVOTION ABOVE I HAVE IDENTIFIED . . .

The lie I believe:

The truth I now receive:

☐ ☐ ☐ I practiced healthy self-talk today (one to three times).

My key personal statement is:

☐ ☐ ☐ I have repeated that message at least three times today.

☐ I have written my personal statement above on an index card or in a journal that I can continue to read if I need renewal in this area.

Nourish Your Body—The Big C

Cancer. I hate that word. More specifically, I hate the disease. In the mid-1970s, I was a new registered nurse and spent one summer on the oncology floor of a large Seattle medical center. And in those short three months, I watched at least a dozen patients between the ages of eight and forty die of cancer. I've lost three of four grandparents to the dreaded disease, and my mother had a full mastectomy twenty-three years ago when she was my exact age today. Most people have wondered now and then if a headache, lump, or some odd symptom could possibly be cancer.

According to data from the American Cancer Society, 63 percent of cancer deaths are caused by smoking, poor diet, physical inactivity, or obesity. Hopefully that fact is just one more good motivation to change our lifestyles. Amazingly, simple and consistent changes can decrease your risk in big ways. For example, simply eating two servings of fruits and three of vegetables each day can reduce your risk of cancer. Additionally, five thirty-minute exercise sessions per week can also increase your protection.

For years scientists have postulated that a healthy immune system may fight cancer on its own without the individual even knowing it. So, doing all you can to stay healthy is essential. Naturopath Dr. Mark Stengler recommends, in addition to consistently eating nutrient-dense foods, the following supplements as especially helpful in fighting cancer:

Folic acid—Found in studies to reduce the risk of breast cancer by 45 percent. Some studies also link folic acid intake to a decreased risk of colon cancer. The usual recommended dosage is four hundred micrograms (mcg) a day. And it is also thought that while a glass or two of wine per day may increase breast cancer risk, taking adequate folic acid may wipe out that risk.

Calcium—According to a study by the American Cancer Society, calcium supplementation decreased colon cancer risk by 30 percent. The usual recommended dosage is 1,000–1,200 mg per day.

Vitamin D—Some studies are suggesting that sufficient vitamin D may cut breast cancer risk by up to 50 percent, and when taken in combination with calcium, it appears to be protective against cancers such as prostate, colon, and others by 60 percent. To get this benefit, one must take a much higher dose than the currently recommended 200–400 international units (IU) and instead take 1,000 IU per day.

DAILY JOURNAL & LOG

My unhealthy habit(s) is diminishing and my new habits are increasing in the following ways:

Nutrition and Fat Management

I ate for maximum energy and health today in the following ways:

- ☐ By drinking 4 to 6 ounces of water most waking hours.
- ☐ By eating protein and/or fiber at breakfast.
- ☐ By eating 3 to 4 vegetables.
- ☐ By eating 2 to 3 servings of fruits, whole grains, or nuts.
- ☐ By eating 5 to 6 snacks or small meals.
- ☐ By eating less from bags and boxes.
- ☐ By eating only when I was hungry.
- ☐ By eating 20 to 50 percent less food than usual in the last 4 hours of the day.
- ☐ By eating no more than 10 percent "empty" calories.

Rest and Regeneration

Last night I slept ____________ hours.

The quality of my sleep was: __________________

Tonight I will ________________________________ to ensure I get quality rest.

Today I managed my stress by:

Tomorrow I will unwind and relax by:

☐ I practiced deep breathing today for relaxation and health.

Fitness

☐ Today I did my minimum 10 minutes of exercise.

I exceeded the minimum by ______________________

Tomorrow I will improve or maintain my fitness by:

Thoughts for Today

day 26

Nourish Your Spirit—Rooted, Built Up, and Strengthened

> So then, just as you received Christ Jesus as Lord, continue to live in him, rooted and built up in him, strengthened in the faith as you were taught, and overflowing with thankfulness.
>
> Colossians 2:6–7

Our home away from home in Lugano sits right next to an old, tree-filled little park. One day I heard several men's voices in the park yelling at each other in Italian. Then an hour later I kept hearing a helicopter overhead coming and going again and again. Of course it roused my curiosity, so I walked out into my yard and looked up only to see a gigantic tree being flown away. Over the course of the afternoon, four such trees disappeared from our park. I'm sure I'll never know why.

When I took my dog for a walk the next day, I was surprised to see the huge stubby trunks of those trees still solidly in the ground, their gigantic old roots digging into the surrounding earth. They could cut their tops off, but the roots remained as solid as ever. It took them years to grow that big and strong, and it would take some serious effort to move them now.

Those are the kind of roots the Lord wants us to have in the person of Jesus. Roots so deep and strong that even in the midst of great calamity, they cling powerfully and are impossible to pull up. God has given us all we need to be rooted, built up, and strengthened in our faith. If we keep our eyes on Christ, our mind on his Word, and our heart connected in love to both God and others, we are unshakeable.

But, like newly planted saplings, it takes time to grow strong, deep roots. We need the instruction and fellowship of more mature believers to protect us until we are mature and able to withstand the changing seasons of life. Three of the four trees that were removed had intertwined roots. It was difficult to tell which root belonged to which tree. That is how we need to be rooted to Christ and to each other. It is what strengthens us for the journey of life.

Like changing habits, growing in the Lord takes time. A fleeting moment of motivation does not keep us going, but deep love and commitment to Christ do. Invest the time it takes to change your mind and change your habits (especially your spiritual ones), for it will truly change your life. A life deeply rooted in Christ can be easily evidenced by the overflowing thankfulness it produces.

Prayer

Dear Lord, I need and want to be deeply rooted in you, built up and strong for this journey. I know that I need to make time with you and in your Word my greatest priority, and yet some days life just gets in the way. Please help me to find quiet moments in each day to connect meaningfully with you. Help me choose the best from all the good so that I will overflow with thankfulness in my heart for you and all you have done. In Jesus's name, amen.

FROM THE DEVOTION ABOVE I HAVE IDENTIFIED . . .

The lie I believe:

The truth I now receive:

☐ ☐ ☐ I practiced healthy self-talk today (one to three times).

My key personal statement is:

☐ ☐ ☐ I have repeated that message at least three times today.

☐ I have written my personal statement above on an index card or in a journal that I can continue to read if I need renewal in this area.

Nourish Your Body—Our Wonderful Sense of Sight

With the exception of gray hair—which is easily hidden with a little hair color—my first real sign of aging came through my eyes. No matter how young you may look on the outside, it's easy to guess your age if you are holding your menu at a restaurant at arm's length! Those are usually the folks in their early forties who have not yet given in to having reading glasses always nearby.

But farsightedness is not the only challenge facing our eyesight. Decades of inadequate nutrition may finally catch up with you in the area of your vision. Like all our body parts, our eyes need optimum nutrition to function properly. We also need to protect them environmentally from ultraviolet rays by wearing UV sunglasses whenever we are out in sunlight.

In addition to a daily intake of a variety of fruits and vegetables, several supplements can make a big difference in your eye function if taken consistently. Bilberry is a popular herb that is packed with potent antioxidants that reduce cellular damage and improve circulation through the smallest capillaries as well as strengthen the tiny vessel walls. Improved circulation allows valuable nutrients to flow to areas such as the retina. The recommended dosage is 160 milligrams twice daily. Eating blueberries regularly can also promote eye health.

Other supplements helpful in dealing with vision include vitamin C, vitamin E, zinc, and ginkgo biloba. Ginkgo is especially effective in treating macular degeneration, diabetic retinopathy, and cataracts.

DAILY JOURNAL & LOG

My unhealthy habit(s) is diminishing and my new habits are increasing in the following ways:

Nutrition and Fat Management

I ate for maximum energy and health today in the following ways:

- ☐ By drinking 4 to 6 ounces of water most waking hours.
- ☐ By eating protein and/or fiber at breakfast.
- ☐ By eating 3 to 4 vegetables.
- ☐ By eating 2 to 3 servings of fruits, whole grains, or nuts.
- ☐ By eating 5 to 6 snacks or small meals.
- ☐ By eating less from bags and boxes.
- ☐ By eating only when I was hungry.
- ☐ By eating 20 to 50 percent less food than usual in the last 4 hours of the day.
- ☐ By eating no more than 10 percent "empty" calories.

Rest and Regeneration

Last night I slept ____________ hours.

The quality of my sleep was: ________________

Tonight I will ______________________________ to ensure I get quality rest.

Today I managed my stress by:

Tomorrow I will unwind and relax by:

☐ I practiced deep breathing today for relaxation and health.

Fitness

☐ Today I did my minimum 10 minutes of exercise.

I exceeded the minimum by _____________________

Tomorrow I will improve or maintain my fitness by:

Thoughts for Today

day 27

Nourish Your Spirit—According to His Will

> This is the confidence we have in approaching God: that if we ask anything according to his will, he hears us. And if we know that he hears us—whatever we ask—we know that we have what we asked of him.
>
> 1 John 5:14–15

Have you ever called out to God over and over, asking him for something really important to you and feeling like he isn't hearing you? Sheri felt that way. She and her husband, John, had been struggling with money issues for as long as she could remember. And for as long as she remembered, Sheri had been praying for a blessing from above. She didn't want to be rich; she simply did not want to live in constant financial and emotional stress. Why was God not answering their prayers?

When we are in a life struggle, it is often hard to see things accurately. In Sheri's case, she was asking for God to deliver her and John from a series of really bad choices. They had spent more money than they made for a long time, and finally the credit had run out and they were unable to sustain their lifestyle. The focus of their prayer was always asking God to provide them money to pay off their debt. But in reality, they had not done their part in being obedient to God's principles in this area of their life. They needed to stop spending and perhaps even sell those things they really could not afford in the first place. They needed to take responsibility and live according to God's precepts. If they had prayed for wisdom, God would have given them wisdom from his Word to manage their money in accordance with his will. If they had asked for favor in finding a buyer for an expensive car or to downsize their home, God may have provided one. I cannot second-guess God, but it is my understanding from Scripture and my own difficult life experiences that God cares more about our character and growth than our comfort. This is true in every dimension of our lives.

Don't get me wrong. I'm not saying that our obedience to God insulates us from life's blows. As it says in Matthew 5:45: "He causes his sun to rise on the evil and the good, and sends rain on the righteous and the unrighteous." But our obedience *is* God's will. So when we pray, we must know God's Word and pray in accordance with it. God cannot answer a prayer that reinforces our disobedient behavior. If you are looking for answers in your life, look first to God's truth in the Bible. Then pray for him to help you obey and live according to it.

However we live, we reap what we sow. At times in our desperation, God in his incredible mercy may give us a moment of reprieve despite our disobedience. But I sense from my own life, this happens to give me another chance to follow his plans rather than my own. God wants to bless us in accordance with his will. When our lifestyles in any area are not in keeping with his perfect principles, distress, disharmony, and disease can follow. Seek his truth and then pray in great confidence. He will answer and supply your need.

Prayer

Dear Lord, thank you for providing me all I need to know to live in accordance with your will within your Word. Forgive me for not always taking the time to read and apply what you have already provided me in the way of instruction. I do desire to follow you in every area of my life. I have not always reaped a healthy harvest. Please give me the strength, wisdom, and conviction to choose your way. In Jesus's name, amen.

FROM THE DEVOTION ABOVE I HAVE IDENTIFIED . . .

The lie I believe:

The truth I now receive:

☐ ☐ ☐ I practiced healthy self-talk today (one to three times).

My key personal statement is:

☐ ☐ ☐ I have repeated that message at least three times today.

☐ I have written my personal statement above on an index card or in a journal that I can continue to read if I need renewal in this area.

Nourish Your Body—Our Top Ten Supplement List

I was blessed to spend almost four years cohosting a San Diego health radio show with dynamic and brilliant naturopath Mark Stengler. Often listeners would ask us about the supplements we felt were most universally needed by people. As a result, Dr. Stengler created the following list.

#1 High-Potency Vitamin-Mineral Complex. Busy lifestyles, poor eating habits, and the diminished quality of our food makes supplementation a necessity in this day and age. The foundation of our program (always secondary to good eating) is a quality vitamin-mineral complex ideally taken in at least two doses for maximum absorption. Capsule and liquid formulas ensure your supplement is absorbed. Some tablets can absorb well; to be sure, put it in a glass of water with one teaspoon of vinegar and see how it breaks down in thirty to sixty minutes with only gentle stirring.

#2 Super Green Foods. Super green foods such as wheat grass, barley grass, alfalfa, spirulina, chlorella, and kelp are excellent sources of real foods that are very high in antioxidant nutrition. They are a great way to help add alkaline to your diet and also enhance your health in many other ways including detoxification, increased immune function, blood sugar stabilization, and increased energy. Despite their plant base, super green foods are a fair source of protein and an excellent source of chlorophyll, which is a great antioxidant and may have some cancer prevention properties.

#3 Essential Fatty Acids. Want to have a sharp mind and great skin? The essential fatty acid omega-3 is a nutrient you need on a daily basis. Because we have limited food sources that are high in omega-3 (such as wild salmon, sardines, walnuts, and flaxseeds), it is unrealistic for most people to get adequate amounts in their daily diets. (Only salmon can supply a sufficient amount of omega-3 to meet the daily requirement in one serving. All the other foods have considerably less and must be eaten consistently and in larger quantities.) Therefore, supplementation is essential. It is essential to use supplements that have been processed to remove the mercury or other heavy metals and to maintain freshness, since fish oil can become rancid if not properly manufactured and stored. My two favorites are Coromega and Nordic Naturals. Neither tastes fishy and both are excellent quality. If you have trouble finding them in your local health food store, I always offer specials on my website.

#4 Vitamin C. While most animals can manufacture their own vitamin C, humans need to get it in their diets. A potent antioxidant with great immunity boosting effects, it also has some of its own unique characteristics. For example, vitamin C is required for the production of collagen, it strengthens capillaries, and it may be helpful for those who bruise easily. It also is very helpful in dealing with arthritis because of its anti-inflammatory properties. As a cancer fighting agent, vitamin C protects the genetic material in cells (DNA) from damage. The average person can take at least two thousand milligrams per day in divided doses. For those with arthritis and some other health complaints, even more may be recommended.

#5 Garlic. This is one of the most researched herbs in the world, with extraordinary attributes both as a food and supplement. Its main medicinal benefits include cardiovascular protection, improved cholesterol levels, lowered blood pressure, diminished blood clotting, improved circulation, and protection against cancer and infectious diseases.

#6 Calcium/Magnesium. Calcium is required by every cell of your body for a variety of actions including muscle contraction, healthy nerves, cell division, and the release of neurotransmitters that scoot between nerve cells, not to mention healthy bones and teeth. Only 10 percent of adults get enough calcium each day. And most children are falling short as well. Caffeine, alcohol, and sugar all promote urinary excretion of calcium. Hormone imbalances and poor digestive function can also contribute to calcium deficiency. From eight years old to eighty, most people need at least 1,000 mg a day of good quality calcium, which is best absorbed in 500 mg doses with at least 250 mg of magnesium.

#7 Vitamin E. Vitamin E is found in the fats of most vegetables and grains, but processing foods destroys this vital nutrient that has both antioxidant properties as well as important support to the nervous system, muscle function, and overall healing. People with diseases such as diabetes, Parkinson's disease, fibrocystic breast syndrome, and multiple sclerosis should have extra E supplementation. The average adult should take 400 IU daily. The best source is a mixed vitamin E that contains a blend of vitamin compounds known as astocopherols and tocotrienols—take 200 to 400 IU daily.

#8 Ginkgo Biloba. This mighty little plant is something I prescribe on a daily basis to treat a wide range of conditions from memory impairment and dizziness to headaches and depression. It has an extraordinary ability to increase circulation to the brain and extremities. Its natural blood-thinning effects are important to the prevention of strokes and heart attacks. I suggest 60 milligrams two to four times per day. For severe cases, like early stage Alzheimer's disease, take 240 to 360 milligrams daily.

#9 Green Tea. With about half the amount of caffeine as coffee, green tea provides a reasonable energy boost without the sharp ups and downs of coffee and its calcium-robbing effects. It is a great antioxidant and anti-cancer agent that also helps the liver with detoxification, which is essential for balancing hormones and cleansing the body of many forms of toxins. Preliminary research shows that green tea can help stabilize blood sugar and thus indirectly promote weight loss by preventing insulin spikes. Green tea extract is available in liquid and capsule forms and a convenient way to get a sufficient dosage in one serving.

#10 Milk Thistle. Most people in America have significant toxins in their bodies, and their livers are overburdened. Our bodies are not equipped to deal with the staggering amount of chemicals that bombard us on a daily basis. Milk thistle is a potent herb that works specifically in the protection and revitalization of our liver and kidney cells. It is also shown to lower glucose levels in those with diabetes and stimulates good digestion of fats as well as improves elimination. I recommend one 250-milligram capsule three times a day.

DAILY JOURNAL & LOG

My unhealthy habit(s) is diminishing and my new habits are increasing in the following ways:

Nutrition and Fat Management

I ate for maximum energy and health today in the following ways:

- ☐ By drinking 4 to 6 ounces of water most waking hours.
- ☐ By eating protein and/or fiber at breakfast.
- ☐ By eating 3 to 4 vegetables.
- ☐ By eating 2 to 3 servings of fruits, whole grains, or nuts.
- ☐ By eating 5 to 6 snacks or small meals.
- ☐ By eating less from bags and boxes.

☐ By eating only when I was hungry.

☐ By eating 20 to 50 percent less food than usual in the last 4 hours of the day.

☐ By eating no more than 10 percent "empty" calories.

Rest and Regeneration

Last night I slept ____________ hours.

The quality of my sleep was: _________________

Tonight I will ______________________________ to ensure I get quality rest.

Today I managed my stress by:

Tomorrow I will unwind and relax by:

☐ I practiced deep breathing today for relaxation and health.

Fitness

☐ Today I did my minimum 10 minutes of exercise.

I exceeded the minimum by _____________________

Tomorrow I will improve or maintain my fitness by:

Thoughts for Today

day 28

Nourish Your Spirit—Created for Good Works

> For we are God's workmanship, created in Christ Jesus to do good works, which God prepared in advance for us to do.
>
> Ephesians 2:10

Years ago when our pastor went on vacation, he asked an older gentleman in his midseventies to preach in his absence. From the moment the guest preacher opened his mouth, the joy of the Lord was evident in his life. He actually spoke with the biggest smile on his face I'd ever seen. He shared that after decades of ministry he and his bride of over fifty years get up each day and say "Good morning, Lord. We're here reporting for duty once again. Thanks for another day of life to serve you. What do you have in mind for us today, Lord?" What an incredible perspective.

What is holding you back from doing the good works God created you to do? Does your health slow you down? Do you feel inadequate because you have allowed a bad habit to consume you and have lost all your confidence that God even wants to use you? No matter what is holding you back, God's plan and purpose, prepared in advance for you, is to work for his glory.

Yesterday is gone. Today is a fresh, clean slate, and God has prepared opportunities for you to make a difference for eternity . . . today. We are saved by grace, not because of works (Eph. 2:8–9), but now that we have been given this magnificent gift, the Lord wants us to produce good works. Once we have fulfilled our ultimate purpose of having a relationship with God through Christ, our next purpose (prepared in advance) is to do good works—that is, impact other lives for eternity.

It doesn't matter where you work, if you're a stay-at-home mom, if you're retired, or even if you're an invalid. God will supply opportunities every day for you to do good works that bring him glory. If we just slow down and really notice what is going on around us, we'd be amazed at the possibilities. Good works are not limited to the ministry that you become involved with at church, the tithe you pay, or the missions you support. It is much more than that.

Did you notice the sadness in the clerk's face at the grocery store? Could you hear your friend's need to talk something out when she called as you were running out the door? Does someone need prayer? Sometimes as I am driving I notice sad- or angry-looking people on the street or in their cars—perhaps even angry if I've made a little driving mistake! Often I feel prompted to pray for that person. I'm not sure of their need, but God certainly is. And I will never know the benefit of those prayers; at least not before heaven. Divine appointments and opportunities to do good works cross our path every day; let's not miss them!

Prayer

> Our awesome God, thank you for the free gift of eternal life that has nothing to do with how good I am or the good things that I do. I know nothing I do can earn my way to heaven. Yet, I am thankful that you give me a purpose as your child to make a difference in the lives of others by doing good works that build up others in the faith or draw people to you. Help me to not miss the opportunities you have prepared in advance for me. Forgive me for the times I have missed those divine appointments. In Jesus's name I pray, amen.

FROM THE DEVOTION ABOVE I HAVE IDENTIFIED . . .

The lie I believe:

The truth I now receive:

☐ ☐ ☐ I practiced healthy self-talk today (one to three times).

My key personal statement is:

☐ ☐ ☐ I have repeated that message at least three times today.

☐ I have written my personal statement above on an index card or in a journal that I can continue to read if I need renewal in this area.

Nourish Your Body—Thyroid News You Can Use

While most people who are overweight are simply eating too much and moving too little, there is an increasing population of women in their forties who have underactive thyroids that don't show up on traditional blood tests for TSH (thyroid stimulating hormone) levels.

According to pharmacist Amanda Edleman, there are more than twenty million people in the United States suffering from hypothyroidism.[1] In addition, 30 percent of women over fifty have significant symptoms of low thyroid despite normal blood tests. If left untreated, symptoms will increase and include (1) gaining weight without overeating; (2) persistent fatigue or even exhaustion; (3) irritability; (4) frequently feeling cold; (5) unexplained depression or anxiety; (6) mental fogginess; (7) out-of-the-ordinary dry skin or hair; (8) low libido; (9) sleep difficulties; (10) unexplainable aches and pains; and more.

If you answer yes to two or more of the symptoms above, you should consider having your thyroid tested comprehensively. According to Edleman, standard thyroid tests are not sufficient to detect all hypothyroid conditions. A saliva test is ideal as it can measure "free or available" thyroid hormones in the body. This type of testing is much more sensitive to detecting low or insufficient levels of thyroid hormones. Unfortunately, many traditional medical doctors rely only on blood tests. At the very least, ask your doctor to include T3 and T4 levels if he or she insists on a blood test. Also, you can get a saliva test kit from many health food stores and send it in for testing. However, doing it this way may not be covered by insurance—so try to work with your own doctor first. Additionally, once results are in, you must have a doctor prescribe thyroid medication if it is needed. I highly recommend a natural thyroid product—Armor Thyroid—in lieu of synthetic brands. I have had hypothyroidism for over ten years and maintained a lean body by eating right, exercising, and taking the appropriate thyroid replacement therapy.

DAILY JOURNAL & LOG

My unhealthy habit(s) is diminishing and my new habits are increasing in the following ways:

Nutrition and Fat Management

I ate for maximum energy and health today in the following ways:

- ☐ By drinking 4 to 6 ounces of water most waking hours.
- ☐ By eating protein and/or fiber at breakfast.
- ☐ By eating 3 to 4 vegetables.
- ☐ By eating 2 to 3 servings of fruits, whole grains, or nuts.
- ☐ By eating 5 to 6 snacks or small meals.

- ☐ By eating less from bags and boxes.
- ☐ By eating only when I was hungry.
- ☐ By eating 20 to 50 percent less food than usual in the last 4 hours of the day.
- ☐ By eating no more than 10 percent "empty" calories.

Rest and Regeneration

Last night I slept ____________ hours.

The quality of my sleep was: _________________

Tonight I will ______________________________ to ensure I get quality rest.

Today I managed my stress by:

Tomorrow I will unwind and relax by:

- ☐ I practiced deep breathing today for relaxation and health.

Fitness

- ☐ Today I did my minimum 10 minutes of exercise.

I exceeded the minimum by _____________________

Tomorrow I will improve or maintain my fitness by:

Thoughts for Today

day 29

Nourish Your Spirit—Reality 24/7

> O Lord, you have searched me
> and you know me.
> You know when I sit and when I rise;
> you perceive my thoughts from afar.
> You discern my going out and my lying down;
> you are familiar with all my ways.
> Before a word is on my tongue
> you know it completely, O Lord.
>
> Psalm 139:1–4

Imagine sitting down to watch television and realizing that the last twenty-four hours of your life has been recorded and broadcast without you knowing it. Think about the last day. Do you consider your time well spent? Did you celebrate the crisp morning air and praise God for his creation? Did you miss the heart cry of a friend over the whirl of the blender? Was there a chance for you to share the hope of the gospel with someone who is desperately seeking? How did you honor God with your body, soul, and spirit yesterday? What things would make you cringe if you had to watch them as a rerun?

As you already know, your loving Father in heaven watches you on a "live feed" all the time. He doesn't watch in judgment only but in a way only a loving Father can. He sees all of you—your brokenness, your dreams, your struggles—and he counts you worthy if you believe you are forgiven by the blood of Christ. He wants all of you, as his worthy heir.

God knows that this fast-paced life with all the noise and distractions makes it easy to lose touch with our real purpose. But he doesn't want our excuses. He wants our total surrender, not out of fear that he will broadcast our failures, but out of love for what he has already done for us.

In order to look back at each day with great joy and a sense that we have fulfilled our purpose, we must be fully focused on the value of each moment. God's purpose is not so much about what grand things we accomplish in the future. As I wrote earlier at the beginning of this book, God's purpose is for this very moment . . . for the sixty seconds in each minute and the sixty minutes in each hour. To live with purpose we must invest in this very moment. If we eat, drink, speak, rest, relate, work, and worship with this simple principle in mind, God is glorified and we grow more and more into the likeness of Christ.

Prayer

Father God, I know your loving eyes are always on me; your Holy Spirit always available to guide me. Thank you for this. I am sure at times I break your heart with my self-centered actions. Please forgive me for my selfishness and help me to be more mindful of how I use each minute of life you have given me. I pray this in Jesus's precious name, amen.

FROM THE DEVOTION ABOVE I HAVE IDENTIFIED . . .

The lie I believe:

The truth I now receive:

☐ ☐ ☐ I practiced healthy self-talk today (one to three times).

My key personal statement is:

☐ ☐ ☐ I have repeated that message at least three times today.

☐ I have written my personal statement above on an index card or in a journal that I can continue to read if I need renewal in this area.

Nourish Your Body—Outsmarting Osteoporosis

I have a confession. Despite my medical and fitness experience, I have often ignored certain health concerns—like osteoporosis. I assumed that my decades of exercise and good nutrition would certainly insulate me from this "old lady" disease. But I'm not burying my head in the sand anymore. Despite my considerable strength and fitness for my age, I cannot ignore the statistics. One out of two women over fifty will have an osteoporosis-related fracture in their lifetime. And while women are more prone to osteoporosis, men are susceptible as well. Since it is very difficult to reverse bone loss, it makes sense to prevent it!

Bone is living tissue that is constantly breaking down and reforming. It is estimated that we have a completely new skeleton every seven years. But if we're not eating the right nutrients and getting enough exercise, the frame we will have tomorrow will be inferior to the one we have today. Osteoporosis means "porous bone." It begins without signs or symptoms, but over time we find ourselves shrinking. Some people with a severe condition can actually fracture a bone simply by bumping into something.

There are many factors that contribute to osteoporosis beyond the normal changes associated with menopause in women. Some of these include family history; no full-term pregnancies; late menses or irregular periods; thin or small body frame; diabetes; eating disorders; kidney or liver disease; many medications, including excessive thyroid hormone replacement; high caffeine, sugar, or alcohol consumption; poor gastric absorption; smoking; inactivity; and low hormone levels.

According to naturopathic doctor Mark Stengler, if low hormones and diminished bone density are both present, natural progesterone either used by itself or in addition to bioidentical estrogen is recommended to treat osteoporosis. Researchers have also found an interesting connection between an imbalanced immune system and bone loss—one more reason to eat and live for optimal health.

There are several ways to stimulate strong bones and prevent osteoporosis. They include regular weight bearing and strength training exercise; excellent nutrition, including lots of plant foods to promote alkalinity in the body, essential fats, and sufficient protein but less from animal sources; the reduction of stress; and bone-specific supplements.

For supplementation, Dr. Stengler recommends 1,200 mg of calcium citrate, aspartate, or gluconate per day taken in divided doses. Additionally, 500 mg of magnesium are essential to ensure calcium absorption. Lastly, vitamin D at 400 to 1,200 IU per day and vitamin K at 150 to 500 mg per day help ensure strong, healthy bones.

DAILY JOURNAL & LOG

My unhealthy habit(s) is diminishing and my new habits are increasing in the following ways:

Nutrition and Fat Management

I ate for maximum energy and health today in the following ways:

- ☐ By drinking 4 to 6 ounces of water most waking hours.
- ☐ By eating protein and/or fiber at breakfast.
- ☐ By eating 3 to 4 vegetables.

☐ By eating 2 to 3 servings of fruits, whole grains, or nuts.

☐ By eating 5 to 6 snacks or small meals.

☐ By eating less from bags and boxes.

☐ By eating only when I was hungry.

☐ By eating 20 to 50 percent less food than usual in the last 4 hours of the day.

☐ By eating no more than 10 percent "empty" calories.

Rest and Regeneration

Last night I slept ____________ hours.

The quality of my sleep was: _________________

Tonight I will ______________________________ to ensure I get quality rest.

Today I managed my stress by:

Tomorrow I will unwind and relax by:

☐ I practiced deep breathing today for relaxation and health.

Fitness

☐ Today I did my minimum 10 minutes of exercise.

I exceeded the minimum by _____________________

Tomorrow I will improve or maintain my fitness by:

Thoughts for Today

day 30

Nourish Your Spirit—Difficult Choice

> For to me, to live is Christ and to die is gain. If I am to go on living in the body, this will mean fruitful labor for me. Yet what shall I choose? I do not know!
>
> Philippians 1:21–22

When we first moved to Europe, we could not find a church service in English nearby, so we spent many Sundays sitting out on our porch and looking out at the spectacular foothills of the Alps and the lake as we talked about God, prayed, and often shared communion as a family. One Sunday, my husband, Lew, was on a business trip, so my eleven-year-old, Jesse, and I had "church" on our own. As we sat looking out at the sky and talking about how beautifully God created our new home, I said to Jesse, "It's like heaven on earth here." Then I asked him if he was excited to go to heaven one day, to which he replied, "Yes, I know it will be great, but I want to be married and be a dad first." I was deeply touched because I know that Jesse's love for Lew and their special bond has made him want to be a father. Jesse is our grandson whom we've adopted and is an incredible gift to Lew and me as we never had children together. Yet, despite the warm fuzzy moment, I didn't want Jesse to miss the important reality that heaven and eternity with God can never be surpassed by any experience here on earth, so I decided to share an illustration I thought he would understand.

"Jesse, do you remember the little carnival we went to that was by the grocery store when you were little?" "Sure, Mom," he replied. "Which did you like better, the little carnival or Disneyland?" I asked. "Duh . . . Disneyland, of course!" he answered with his incredulous eleven-year-old attitude. "Well, Jess . . . this is the thing. Just like Disneyland is way, way better than the carnival, heaven is way, way better than anything we will ever have here on earth, even being a husband or a dad. Do you believe that?" "Uh-huh," he slowly answered and then after a long pause blurted out, "But I still want to be a dad!"

Just like Jesse, most of us cling to the things of this world that we know because we can barely get our minds around the immensity of heaven, not to mention letting go of life as we know it and of those we love. If we completely understood, we would be able to honestly exclaim in concert with the apostle Paul, "To me, to live is Christ and to die is gain. What shall I choose?"

One day when we reach heaven, I'm sure it will finally hit us how ridiculous we were to cling so tightly to the things of this world when all that we really want, need, and desire is fully realized in heaven.

Prayer

Heavenly Father, I want to know Jesus in such a powerful way that I can say with Paul, "To live is Christ, to die is gain." I know that my faith must grow for that to become my true heart's cry. Please help me to release my attachment to the things of this world. Like Paul, I want to live and serve you for as many days as you give me. But I also want to welcome my journey home to you without fear or hesitation, knowing that to be apart from the body is to be present with you, Lord. Let me live each day to the fullest to your glory until you call me home. In Jesus's name, amen.

FROM THE DEVOTION ABOVE I HAVE IDENTIFIED . . .

The lie I believe:

The truth I now receive:

☐ ☐ ☐ I practiced healthy self-talk today (one to three times).

My key personal statement is:

☐ ☐ ☐ I have repeated that message at least three times today.

☐ I have written my personal statement above on an index card or in a journal that I can continue to read if I need renewal in this area.

Nourish Your Body—Top Ten Fruits and Vegetables

The most common fruits eaten regularly by Americans are bananas and apples. Both are full of excellent nutrition. But your body needs a variety of nutrients. And if you find it difficult to get in the recommended two to three servings per day, try to pick at least one from the top ten list below. These fruits supply the highest quantity of carotenoids, folic acid, potassium, vitamin C, and fiber:

1. Guava
2. Blueberries
3. Watermelon
4. Grapefruit (pink or red)
5. Kiwi
6. Papaya
7. Cantaloupe
8. Apricots (dried)
9. Oranges
10. Strawberries

As you might guess, the top two veggies that Americans eat are potatoes (in the form of French fries) and tomatoes (in the form of ketchup). It's time to move onward and upward beyond even carrots and green beans to the top ten list of veggies that have the highest quantity of carotenoids, folic acid, potassium, vitamin C, and fiber, plus calcium:

1. Collard greens
2. Spinach
3. Kale
4. Swiss chard
5. Red pepper
6. Sweet potatoes
7. Pumpkin (canned)
8. Carrots
9. Broccoli
10. Okra

Fresh produce tastes wonderful when in season, so experiment with all the color, crunch, and leafy greens. Don't forget to check the frozen section in the grocery store when fresh produce is not available. Frozen fruits and vegetables are preserved at the peak of their nutritional value, and some contain just as many nutrients as fresh produce—sometimes more, depending on how long the fresh ones have sat on display or in a refrigerator. And canned is better than nothing. (Note: many products have added sugar, so buy unsweetened frozen and canned fruits. Also, rinse canned vegetables to reduce the sodium content.)

DAILY JOURNAL & LOG

My unhealthy habit(s) is diminishing and my new habits are increasing in the following ways:

Nutrition and Fat Management

I ate for maximum energy and health today in the following ways:

- ☐ By drinking 4 to 6 ounces of water most waking hours.
- ☐ By eating protein and/or fiber at breakfast.
- ☐ By eating 3 to 4 vegetables.
- ☐ By eating 2 to 3 servings of fruits, whole grains, or nuts.
- ☐ By eating 5 to 6 snacks or small meals.
- ☐ By eating less from bags and boxes.
- ☐ By eating only when I was hungry.
- ☐ By eating 20 to 50 percent less food than usual in the last 4 hours of the day.
- ☐ By eating no more than 10 percent "empty" calories.

Rest and Regeneration

Last night I slept ____________ hours.

The quality of my sleep was: _________________

Tonight I will _______________________________ to ensure I get quality rest.

Today I managed my stress by:

Tomorrow I will unwind and relax by:

☐ I practiced deep breathing today for relaxation and health.

Fitness

☐ Today I did my minimum 10 minutes of exercise.

I exceeded the minimum by ______________________

Tomorrow I will improve or maintain my fitness by:

Thoughts for Today

day 31

Nourish Your Spirit—Ungodly Appetites

> The rabble with them began to crave other food, and again the Israelites started wailing and said, "If only we had meat to eat! We remember the fish we ate in Egypt at no cost—also the cucumbers, melons, leeks, onions and garlic. But now we have lost our appetite; we never see anything but this manna!"
>
> Numbers 11:4–6

Being a slave to a ruthless master would be an unimaginable horror. To labor intensely under the oppressive hand of another who saw you as no better than an animal would crush your spirit and leave you hopeless. This is the kind of life the Israelites lived in Egypt under Pharaoh's rule. In their pain, they cried out to God, who heard their pleas. And God sent Moses to lead them out of captivity to a land flowing with milk and honey. On their journey to freedom, they witness countless miracles that included seeing the Red Sea part to allow them safe passage and then close again just in time for God to allow their enemies to perish. They were miraculously provided fresh water and manna from heaven for food. But despite God's loving protection and generous provision, the people began to grumble. They so craved the food of their captivity that they wanted to return to slavery simply to satisfy their appetites. In fact, they cried out so loudly for meat to eat that God delivered them quail—so much that each person had more than they could consume. In their bondage to their appetites, God's answer to their prayer was not really a blessing, for this is the rest of the story:

> But while the meat was still between their teeth and before it could be consumed, the anger of the LORD burned against the people, and he struck them with a severe plague.
>
> Numbers 11:33

How many of us are slaves to our physical desires? I certainly was for many years. My obsession with food impacted everything I did. When I wasn't thinking about bingeing, I was thinking about dieting. This slavery to food and my eating disorder consumed my life. My focus was not on God. It was on food. I am so thankful that I am blessed to live under the law of grace. Even in my darkest hour, God saw me through with the blood of Christ. Yet, being forgiven is no excuse for bad behavior. God desires us to put him above *all* things. When we cannot control our appetites (whatever they are), we are clearly walking in our flesh and must surrender them to the Lord. It may be a daily battle for a while, but God wants to deliver us from slavery. Call out to him when overwhelming desires for the things you crave consume you, and he will deliver you from bondage.

Prayer

> Heavenly Father, thank you for your love and grace in all things and for providing me with everything I need to live according to your purpose. Please forgive me for craving things above you sometimes. I pray that I would crave you above everything. On this journey to change my mind and my habits to renew my body, soul, and spirit, I pray that you will give me insights and wisdom to address my most important issues. Lord, please expose me to the lies I believe that are

keeping me in bondage. I want to be transformed by the renewing of my mind. Lord, help me take one day at a time and surrender my habits to you. In Jesus's name I pray, amen.

FROM THE DEVOTION ABOVE I HAVE IDENTIFIED . . .

The lie I believe:

The truth I now receive:

☐ ☐ ☐ I practiced healthy self-talk today (one to three times).

My key personal statement is:

☐ ☐ ☐ I have repeated that message at least three times today.

☐ I have written my personal statement above on an index card or in a journal that I can continue to read if I need renewal in this area.

Nourish Your Body—Syndrome X

Some people who have trouble losing weight may have both a genetic and/or possibly lifestyle-generated challenge called Syndrome X or Insulin Resistance Syndrome (IRS).

According to the Centers for Disease Control and Prevention, at least one in four Americans (that's over 47 million) have this body chemistry challenge in which the hormone insulin may double or triple in the bloodstream. IRS is directly associated with high body fat and a sedentary lifestyle. Some experts estimate that more than 140 million adults and 10 million children could be affected.

While genetics may play a role, the primary cause of IRS is lifestyle—too much food and not enough exercise being the most important factors. It has become a silent killer, influencing a wide array of health concerns such as infertility; heart disease; stroke; cancers of the breast, uterus, prostate, and colon; high blood pressure; type-2 diabetes; and perhaps even Alzheimer's disease.

A few key factors can help you determine if you are likely to be at risk for IRS. They include the following: (1) obesity with a body mass index (BMI) higher than 25, or a waist measurement more than 35 inches for women (or 40 inches for men); (2) a sedentary lifestyle; (3) a family or personal history of type-2 diabetes; (4) a history of higher than normal blood sugar; (5) a history of high blood pressure (130/80 or higher); high triglycerides (over 150) or low HDL (under 50 for women); and (6) polycystic ovary syndrome, a condition that reduces a woman's fertility. While it is difficult to conclusively diagnose IRS, a specialized blood sugar test may help your health care professional determine if you are susceptible.

Under normal conditions, our body only needs tiny amounts of insulin to trigger the muscle and liver cells to absorb glucose after food is ingested. But for overweight individuals, the normal mechanism seems to go awry. Body fat, and more specifically belly fat, interferes with this process. For some reason, the immune system treats the excess body fat as an intruder and surrounds it with a team of "disease-fighting" cells that send chemicals into your bloodstream and block insulin's ability to communicate accurately with the cells that should be willing to "accept" the glucose. If this process continues, an individual becomes highly susceptible to acquiring type-2 diabetes.

The solution to Syndrome X is an immediate and consistent lifestyle change that includes a healthy diet with no more than 10 to

15 percent processed foods and refined carbohydrates, and daily adequate exercise. In addition, several supplements can help to balance blood sugar levels in a variety of ways. A teaspoon per day of the spice cinnamon has been shown to decrease cholesterol, reduce blood pressure, and balance blood sugar. Other helpful supplements include chromium, omega-3 fish oil, biotin, ALA, and vanadium.

DAILY JOURNAL & LOG

My unhealthy habit(s) is diminishing and my new habits are increasing in the following ways:

Nutrition and Fat Management

I ate for maximum energy and health today in the following ways:

- ☐ By drinking 4 to 6 ounces of water most waking hours.
- ☐ By eating protein and/or fiber at breakfast.
- ☐ By eating 3 to 4 vegetables.
- ☐ By eating 2 to 3 servings of fruits, whole grains, or nuts.
- ☐ By eating 5 to 6 snacks or small meals.
- ☐ By eating less from bags and boxes.
- ☐ By eating only when I was hungry.
- ☐ By eating 20 to 50 percent less food than usual in the last 4 hours of the day.
- ☐ By eating no more than 10 percent "empty" calories.

Rest and Regeneration

Last night I slept ____________ hours.

The quality of my sleep was: ________________.

Tonight I will ______________________________ to ensure I get quality rest.

Today I managed my stress by:

Tomorrow I will unwind and relax by:

☐ I practiced deep breathing today for relaxation and health.

Fitness

☐ Today I did my minimum 10 minutes of exercise.

I exceeded the minimum by ____________________

Tomorrow I will improve or maintain my fitness by:

Thoughts for Today

day 32

Nourish Your Spirit—Losing Your Marbles

> Be very careful, then, how you live—not as unwise but as wise, making the most of every opportunity, because the days are evil. Therefore do not be foolish, but understand what the Lord's will is.
>
> Ephesians 5:15–17

At 55 years plus 2 months old (as of this writing), I have already lived a whopping 20,147 days. That's 483,528 hours of eating, sleeping, blow-drying, laughing, crying, resting, striving, worshipping, and loving. Wow. I wonder how many more I have left. Only the Lord knows.

I heard a story about a man who figured out a creative way to remind himself each week about the value of his life. After years of putting work and accomplishments ahead of family and God, he decided it was time to get his priorities in order. He realized that he had spent one Saturday too many on things that just didn't matter. One day, he sat down and did a little arithmetic. Since on average, most folks live about 75 years, he figured that he had been allotted 3,900 Saturdays in his lifetime and he was going to live the rest of them to the max! Since he was 55 when he did this math, he figured he had about 1,000 of them left to enjoy. To help him in his endeavor, he went to a local toy store and bought up every marble they had. He took them home and put them inside a large, clear plastic container. Every Saturday, he would take one out and throw it away. He found that by watching the marbles diminish, he could focus better on the more important aspects of his life.

When I heard the story, he had just taken the last marble out of the container. He figured if he could make it until the next Saturday, he was given a little bonus time. I've already used up 2,704 of my Saturdays. I don't mind "losing my marbles" if I feel my life is well invested. It just means that I'm getting that much closer to heaven. But, I do want to be careful and make the most of every opportunity. From the Scripture above, we can see that including the Lord's will into the equation is essential. If this life on earth was simply about coming to a saving faith in Christ, then once that happened, God could simply snatch us up to heaven. But instead he leaves us here on this earth to impact others with his love. There are so many divine appointments that can be missed if we are foolish and self-absorbed in our own plans.

If you don't think the days are evil, you haven't read the papers or turned on the evening news. People need encouragement. People need truth. People need Jesus. If we are encouraging other Christians toward a deeper, more meaningful walk with Christ, giving help to the downtrodden in Jesus's name, loving the unlovely, lifting up the lonely, or sharing the good news, we are making the most of every opportunity. It is in those moments that we become less and he becomes more, and amazingly our personal issues are overshadowed by his heavenly purposes.

Prayer

Lord, help me to know your will for my life each day and to be acutely aware of your heavenly purposes. I pray that I will not simply spend my days but rather invest them for eternity. May you be glorified in the days you give me on this earth. Praise your holy name. Amen.

FROM THE DEVOTION ABOVE I HAVE IDENTIFIED . . .

The lie I believe:

The truth I now receive:

☐ ☐ ☐ I practiced healthy self-talk today (one to three times).

My key personal statement is:

☐ ☐ ☐ I have repeated that message at least three times today.

☐ I have written my personal statement above on an index card or in a journal that I can continue to read if I need renewal in this area.

Nourish Your Body—Healthy Gums . . . Healthy Heart

Taking good care of your gums and teeth also helps protect your entire cardiovascular system. For many years, health professionals have been warning us of the danger of periodontitis (infected gums), which can increase our risk of heart attack and stroke.

Unfortunately, all too often people don't even know their gums are infected. It is important to watch for gums that are red or irritated or that bleed easily. Experts explain that gum disease is caused by plaque buildup, which can be dealt with very effectively with quality brushing and flossing. And of course, annual exams and professional cleaning ensure you are doing a good job.

The theory is that bacteria present in infected gums can come loose and enter your bloodstream through the extremely vascular gum tissue. This same bacteria that irritates gums can travel right into the arteries. Current research shows that risk varies according to the level of gum infection. The worse the infection, the more likely the bacteria is to become blood borne. And because gums tend to bleed, it makes it easier for bacteria to enter the bloodstream. If bacteria reaches the arteries, it can cause inflammation as it does on the gums, potentially causing arterial plaque to accumulate in the arteries. As a result, a hardening and compromised blood flow can result in a heart attack. This same thing can occur in other parts of the body. If blockage occurs in the brain, it can cause a stroke.

A study published in 2004 by the *Journal of Periodontology* reported that periodontitis seems to influence the occurrence and the severity of coronary artery disease and increases the risk of heart attack or stroke. It stated that 91 percent of the people studied who had coronary artery disease (CAD) also had some level of periodontitis.[1]

Carry a toothbrush so you can brush and floss between meals and snacks. And while you are taking a few minutes to do that . . . practice a little healthy self-talk at the same time!

DAILY JOURNAL & LOG

My unhealthy habit(s) is diminishing and my new habits are increasing in the following ways:

Nutrition and Fat Management

I ate for maximum energy and health today in the following ways:

- ☐ By drinking 4 to 6 ounces of water most waking hours.
- ☐ By eating protein and/or fiber at breakfast.
- ☐ By eating 3 to 4 vegetables.
- ☐ By eating 2 to 3 servings of fruits, whole grains, or nuts.
- ☐ By eating 5 to 6 snacks or small meals.
- ☐ By eating less from bags and boxes.
- ☐ By eating only when I was hungry.
- ☐ By eating 20 to 50 percent less food than usual in the last 4 hours of the day.
- ☐ By eating no more than 10 percent "empty" calories.

Rest and Regeneration

Last night I slept ____________ hours.

The quality of my sleep was: _________________

Tonight I will ______________________________ to ensure I get quality rest.

Today I managed my stress by:

Tomorrow I will unwind and relax by:

☐ I practiced deep breathing today for relaxation and health.

Fitness

☐ Today I did my minimum 10 minutes of exercise.

I exceeded the minimum by ______________________

Tomorrow I will improve or maintain my fitness by:

Thoughts for Today

day 33

Nourish Your Spirit—Fulfilling God's Purpose

> With this in mind, we constantly pray for you, that our God may count you worthy of his calling, and that by his power he may fulfill every good purpose of yours and every act prompted by your faith.
>
> 2 Thessalonians 1:11

Does your to-do list seem to grow longer rather than shorter most days? The older we get, the faster time seems to fly. One day, we may look in the mirror and wonder, *Where did all those years go?* Even today, the minutes and hours are slipping away so quickly. You may be wondering, *What have I really accomplished that makes a difference in the bigger scheme of things?* Perhaps the better question is, *What has God accomplished through me?*

When you rolled out of bed this morning, was it your agenda or God's that captured your attention? Have you been sensitive to any divine appointments or opportunities to invest in something of eternal value today? He is ready to "fulfill every good purpose of yours and every act prompted by your faith."

In this fast-paced life with all the noise and distractions, we can lose touch of our real purpose in the mundane details of life—to love each other, to encourage each other in our faith, and to share the hope of the gospel with those who are lost. If we slow down . . . be still . . . cease striving . . . we are more likely to be prompted by our faith.

Paul was constantly praying for the saints in Thessalonica to fulfill their good purposes. Who is praying for you in this way? At the very least, we must pray this prayer for ourselves. Each day holds potential for us to be prompted by faith and to accomplish things of lasting value. But unless we refocus our attention, we may miss God's best for today.

And when we are focused on things with eternal purpose, it is amazing how our weaknesses and problems fade from the forefront of our attention. Take a big breath and redirect your attention from time to time during your day. Ask the Lord to direct your path and prompt you to see the details of your day with spiritual eyes. The phone is ringing . . . I've got to go. It just could be a divine appointment!

Prayer

Father God, I don't want to miss your calling on my life. Open my eyes to see your greater purpose in each day. Forgive me for not always being aware of the opportunities that cross my path. I desire to be your hands and feet in a hurting world. Prompt me to step out in faith and touch lives for your glory. In Jesus's name, amen.

FROM THE DEVOTION ABOVE I HAVE IDENTIFIED . . .

The lie I believe:

The truth I now receive:

☐ ☐ ☐ I practiced healthy self-talk today (one to three times).

My key personal statement is:

☐ ☐ ☐ I have repeated that message at least three times today.

☐ I have written my personal statement above on an index card or in a journal that I can continue to read if I need renewal in this area.

Nourish Your Body—Exercise Your Mind

"Physical activity can make people more mentally alert," says brain researcher Judy Cameron, PhD, of Oregon Health and Science University.[1] Two very interesting studies have strongly supported this statement.

In one of Cameron's studies, monkeys who ran on treadmills grew more blood vessels that supply brain cells with oxygen and blood. Active monkeys navigated a complex maze twice as fast as the unconditioned monkeys. In a mouse study at the University of Wisconsin-Madison, researchers discovered that exercise stimulates production of a substance that prompts neurons to grow and link up.

With advances in medical science, MRI technology can reveal evidence of how brain cells grow. One can witness learning centers in the brain light up and the formation of neural pathways when a person tries something new. Amazing! These kinds of changes and activity can even be evidenced in the elderly.

In addition to exercise, new daily experiences can benefit our brains and expand our minds. By simply breaking some of our routine habits and doing something new, we can increase our brainpower and avoid premature aging of our gray matter. The more you do new things, the more you can benefit.

Here are a few ideas to get you started:

Learn a new language.

Play games like Scrabble.

Do crossword puzzles or other brain-stimulating activities.

Brush your teeth with your opposite hand.

Go to a new grocery store.

Visit a new city.

Try new restaurants with unique ethnic foods.

Walk or run a different route.

DAILY JOURNAL & LOG

My unhealthy habit(s) is diminishing and my new habits are increasing in the following ways:

Nutrition and Fat Management

I ate for maximum energy and health today in the following ways:

- ☐ By drinking 4 to 6 ounces of water most waking hours.
- ☐ By eating protein and/or fiber at breakfast.
- ☐ By eating 3 to 4 vegetables.
- ☐ By eating 2 to 3 servings of fruits, whole grains, or nuts.
- ☐ By eating 5 to 6 snacks or small meals.
- ☐ By eating less from bags and boxes.
- ☐ By eating only when I was hungry.
- ☐ By eating 20 to 50 percent less food than usual in the last 4 hours of the day.
- ☐ By eating no more than 10 percent "empty" calories.

Rest and Regeneration

Last night I slept ____________ hours.

The quality of my sleep was: __________________

Tonight I will ________________________________ to ensure I get quality rest.

Today I managed my stress by:

Tomorrow I will unwind and relax by:

☐ I practiced deep breathing today for relaxation and health.

Fitness

☐ Today I did my minimum 10 minutes of exercise.

I exceeded the minimum by ____________________

Tomorrow I will improve or maintain my fitness by:

Thoughts for Today

day 34

Nourish Your Spirit—Falling Away

> Peter declared, "Even if all fall away, I will not."
>
> "I tell you the truth," Jesus answered, "today—yes, tonight—before the rooster crows twice you yourself will disown me three times."
>
> Mark 14:29–30

There have been times in my spiritual walk when I felt like I was on the top of the mountain with God. My faith was invincible and I could not imagine ever giving in to temptation. Knowing what I knew about God and feeling his strength and power in my life . . . it was simply impossible. That is probably how Peter felt that last night with Jesus. Peter loved Jesus so much, and when Jesus told his disciples that they would *all* fall away from him and be scattered, Peter just could not accept it. And so he emphatically declared otherwise, only to be shattered by Jesus turning to him specifically and telling him that he would disown him three times before dawn. How crushing.

God in his perfect wisdom shows us in Scripture the weaknesses and failings of those who walked in the very presence of Jesus. Can you imagine seeing his miracles firsthand, looking into his eyes, feeling his touch, and still blowing it so badly? Yet, each of the disciples fled for their own sakes that critical night before Jesus's crucifixion. If those who knew him in the flesh were that weak, it is no surprise that we are as well. Jesus knows our weaknesses. He sees our sin and corruption and willingly goes to the cross. He sees us. He knows us. He loves us anyway.

Can you imagine the knife in Peter's heart when he heard the rooster crowing and realized that Jesus was right? He had denied him just as Jesus had said. We all deny Christ in little and big ways. Sometimes when we know God has given us a divine opportunity to share our faith, we do not speak. At other times, if we were to watch ourselves on video, we would see that our actions don't always reveal that we are children of the King. We think we are strong in the Lord and yet we fail again and again to love and honor him as he fully deserves.

When we fall away for a moment or even for a season, how does Jesus respond? He helps us remember our first love. After his resurrection, Jesus appeared to his disciples and prepared breakfast by the lake for them. It always amazes me how Christ meets even our lowly physical needs when more important matters are at hand. After breakfast, Jesus turned his focus to Peter:

> Jesus said to Simon Peter, "Simon, son of Jonah, do you love Me more than these?" He said to Him, "Yes, Lord; You know that I love You." He said to him, "Feed My lambs."
>
> He said to him again a second time, "Simon, son of Jonah, do you love Me?" He said to Him, "Yes, Lord; You know that I love You." He said to him, "Tend My sheep."
>
> He said to him the third time, "Simon, son of Jonah, do you love Me?" Peter was grieved because He said to him the third time, "Do

> you love Me?" And he said to Him, "Lord, You know all things; You know that I love You." Jesus said to him, "Feed My sheep."
>
> John 21:15–17 NASB

Was Jesus that unsure of Peter's love after his betrayal that he needed Peter to tell him three times of his love? Of course not; it was Peter who needed to be secure and reminded that despite his betrayal, his love for Jesus was real and secure. And not only that, Jesus wanted Peter to continue to tend to the new and mature believers he had put into his care.

Don't let the shame of bad behavior or a lapse in your faith keep you from intimate time with Christ and being used for his glory. Do you love him? Do you love him? Do you love him?

Prayer

Oh Jesus, I do love you and I am so grieved when my words and actions do not reveal this. Thank you for showing me in your Word that I am not alone. I pray you will not let the enemy's lies hold me back in shame when I fall away. But, rather I pray that your Holy Spirit will give me faith and assurance that my love for you is real despite my failings and sin. Forgive me for my weakness and strengthen me by your power. Amen.

FROM THE DEVOTION ABOVE I HAVE IDENTIFIED . . .

The lie I believe:

The truth I now receive:

☐ ☐ ☐ I practiced healthy self-talk today (one to three times).

My key personal statement is:

☐ ☐ ☐ I have repeated that message at least three times today.

☐ I have written my personal statement above on an index card or in a journal that I can continue to read if I need renewal in this area.

Nourish Your Body—Burn Fat to the Max!

Burning off fat should be your main objective if you are carrying too much body weight. The scale can't really tell you what you've burned, but you can ensure that most of it is fat if you include regular aerobic activity into your lifestyle—ideally five to six days per week.

As you can see from the graph on the next page, you burn very little fat when you are resting or sedentary (about 5–10 percent). Instead, you are mostly burning the sugar in your bloodstream and stored carbohydrates from you muscles and liver. But when you begin to move aerobically, your body needs to kick into a more efficient and lasting fuel source—fat! Notice on the chart that your fat-burning capacity starts to grow from 5 percent to 50 to 60 percent as you approach thirty minutes of continuous aerobic movement. This reality is why aerobic activity is so essential to fat loss.

Even when you cannot get a full thirty-minute session in, notice how fat metabolism is still much higher than when you don't exercise. Yes, it is ideal to get a few long workouts in each week, but everything counts!

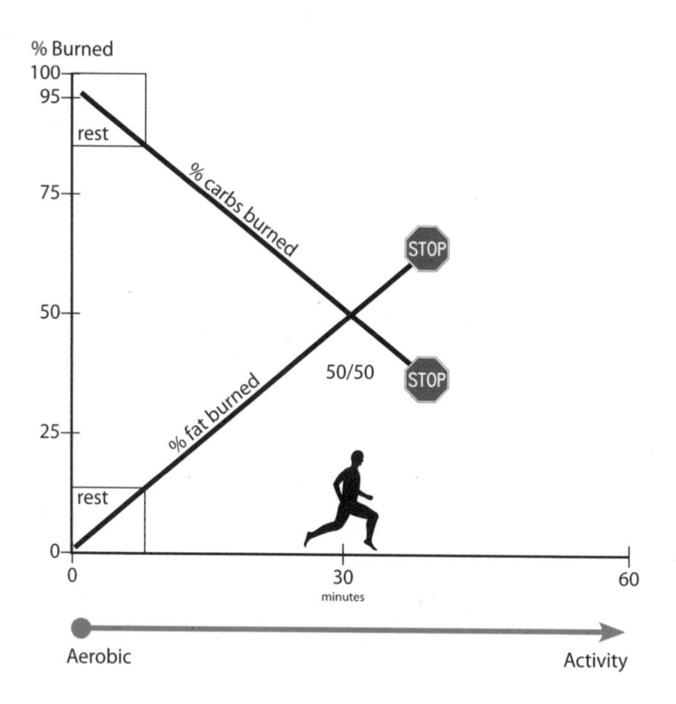

DAILY JOURNAL & LOG

My unhealthy habit(s) is diminishing and my new habits are increasing in the following ways:

Nutrition and Fat Management

I ate for maximum energy and health today in the following ways:

- ☐ By drinking 4 to 6 ounces of water most waking hours.
- ☐ By eating protein and/or fiber at breakfast.
- ☐ By eating 3 to 4 vegetables.

☐ By eating 2 to 3 servings of fruits, whole grains, or nuts.

☐ By eating 5 to 6 snacks or small meals.

☐ By eating less from bags and boxes.

☐ By eating only when I was hungry.

☐ By eating 20 to 50 percent less food than usual in the last 4 hours of the day.

☐ By eating no more than 10 percent "empty" calories.

Rest and Regeneration

Last night I slept ____________ hours.

The quality of my sleep was: _________________

Tonight I will ______________________________ to ensure I get quality rest.

Today I managed my stress by:

Tomorrow I will unwind and relax by:

☐ I practiced deep breathing today for relaxation and health.

Fitness

☐ Today I did my minimum 10 minutes of exercise.

I exceeded the minimum by _____________________

Tomorrow I will improve or maintain my fitness by:

Thoughts for Today

day 35

Nourish Your Spirit—Holy and Self-Controlled

> Therefore, prepare your minds for action; be self-controlled; set your hope fully on the grace to be given you when Jesus Christ is revealed. As obedient children, do not conform to the evil desires you had when you lived in ignorance. But just as he who called you is holy, so be holy in all you do; for it is written: "Be holy, because I am holy."
>
> 1 Peter 1:13–16

In the past two years, I have been on fourteen international flights to and from Europe, in order to fulfill my speaking ministry commitments. While I have no fear of flying, I always say a prayer for safe travel, specifically that our pilots are well rested, alert, and prepared for the journey. On occasion, I observe some of the pilots in the airport and wonder just how they prepare their minds for the responsibility of flying hundreds of people around the world. Can you imagine trusting your life to a pilot who is not willing to take good care of his body, abstain from alcohol, and get a good night's rest before a long flight? Unfortunately, I am sure that happens more often than we'd like to know.

Preparing our minds and being self-controlled is not something we limit to "life and death" areas of life. God calls us to do both in the daily details of our lives. Preparing our minds means that we are able to interpret people and life accurately through the wisdom of God's Word. When we understand his truth and are always ready to respond to circumstances to his glory, we can live with great passion and purpose. Yet, all the knowledge in the world is of little value if we don't apply it to our lives. Moment to moment, we must choose whom we will serve, God or ourselves. In the moment that we choose God, we move from walking in the flesh to walking in the Spirit. And, when we walk in the Spirit, we are empowered with his fruit.

> But the fruit of the Spirit is love, joy, peace, patience, kindness, goodness, faithfulness, gentleness and self-control. Against such things there is no law.
>
> Galatians 5:22–23

All that incredible fruit listed above is an outgrowth of being totally empowered by the Holy Spirit. We don't just get one or two of the fruit listed—we get the entire basket, including self-control. When we are fully equipped in this way, we are unable to sin. But, sadly, in a heartbeat, we can quickly step back into living under our own power.

As obedient children, we live not out of fear of discipline but rather out of deep love and gratitude for God, who saved us in spite of ourselves. We are no longer weak and alone but rather powerful in the Lord. And in his power, we are able to think and act in accordance with his will. We cannot be perfect or holy in our own power, but in his power we are a reflection of Christ.

Prayer

Lord God, please help me to prepare my mind for action each day as I read and study your Word. I pray that you will show me what it means to walk in your Spirit, keeping my mind fixed on your will for my life. Thank you for the grace you give me as I fail to be all you have called me to be. Help me to realize that it is only when I surrender to you that you can use me fully. I want to be holy as you are holy, God. In Jesus's name, amen.

FROM THE DEVOTION ABOVE I HAVE IDENTIFIED . . .

The lie I believe:

The truth I now receive:

☐ ☐ ☐ I practiced healthy self-talk today (one to three times).

My key personal statement is:

☐ ☐ ☐ I have repeated that message at least three times today.

☐ I have written my personal statement above on an index card or in a journal that I can continue to read if I need renewal in this area.

Nourish Your Body—Beans . . . Beans . . . Good for the Body!

Beans are perfect little nutrition packets! Since you need to get great sources of protein and fiber into your diet, a wide assortment of beans can do just that in a heart healthy, energy-increasing way. They supply you with lots of iron, folate, potassium, and calcium and can help lower blood cholesterol and reduce the risk of some types of cancer.

The average person eats about one cup of beans per week. If they give you gas, that's only because you are not eating enough fresh, raw foods to generate the right enzymes to digest them. So, increase those foods and use enzyme supplements so you can add lots of nutritious, fiber-rich beans to your diet every week.

The good news is that canned beans, which are both economical and convenient, are just as nutritious as the ones you cook yourself, with the exception of some with high sodium levels. Read the labels and get those that go light on the sodium whenever possible. Or rinse the beans in a colander to remove much of the salt before adding them to your recipes.

For summer barbeques, I take about four to six varieties of beans and put them in a Crock-Pot with lots of other goodies like grilled onions and peppers. I use a little honey, mustard, and ketchup to spice them up as well. They are always a big hit and can count for one veggie serving as well!

Get creative and toss beans into your salads, spaghetti sauce, or casseroles. Sprinkle healthy, lard-free refried beans with light cheese and use it as a dip with baked corn chips for an extra treat. I like to mix fresh salsa into bean dip to give it more kick both for taste and nutrition. Beans . . . beans . . . are so good for the body!

DAILY JOURNAL & LOG

My unhealthy habit(s) is diminishing and my new habits are increasing in the following ways:

Nutrition and Fat Management

I ate for maximum energy and health today in the following ways:

- ☐ By drinking 4 to 6 ounces of water most waking hours.
- ☐ By eating protein and/or fiber at breakfast.
- ☐ By eating 3 to 4 vegetables.
- ☐ By eating 2 to 3 servings of fruits, whole grains, or nuts.
- ☐ By eating 5 to 6 snacks or small meals.
- ☐ By eating less from bags and boxes.
- ☐ By eating only when I was hungry.
- ☐ By eating 20 to 50 percent less food than usual in the last 4 hours of the day.

☐ By eating no more than 10 percent "empty" calories.

Rest and Regeneration

Last night I slept ____________ hours.

The quality of my sleep was: _________________

Tonight I will ______________________________ to ensure I get quality rest.

Today I managed my stress by:

Tomorrow I will unwind and relax by:

☐ I practiced deep breathing today for relaxation and health.

Fitness

☐ Today I did my minimum 10 minutes of exercise.

I exceeded the minimum by _____________________

Tomorrow I will improve or maintain my fitness by:

Thoughts for Today

day 36

Nourish Your Spirit—No Eye Has Seen

> No eye has seen, no ear has heard, no mind has conceived what God has prepared for those who love him.
>
> 1 Corinthians 2:9

Take a few moments and daydream about how you would spend the perfect week, if time and money were no issue. In this fantasy without limits, your body is healthy and full of vitality; your relationships are intimate and rewarding. You can experience the most amazing things . . . anything you can possibly imagine. Write down somewhere on this page a few of the things that come to mind. Don't hold back . . . the sky is the limit!

Now, let me extend this whimsy and turn your perfect week into five, ten, fifteen, or more years. Gee, since we can do absolutely anything . . . let's make it last forever. The very best you can imagine will never come close to what God has prepared for you if you love him and have received Christ as your personal Savior.

Heaven will be more than we can ever imagine. In his book *90 Minutes in Heaven*, Don Piper shares his almost unbelievable personal experience of spending what he assumes was ninety minutes in heaven. He had been pronounced dead by numerous people before miraculously awaking as a Christian man prayed and sang over him. He was so concerned that no one would believe his story that he shared it only with close friends for many, many years. He figured people would think it was all in his imagination, some kind of a near-death experience. But, as he describes in his book, there was no way he could have been alive without bleeding to death. His death actually stopped the bleeding. When he was "brought back," he was under the immediate care of medics. After much prodding by

Christian friends, Don finally exposed his "sacred secret." Yet as he tried to write about his experience, he kept saying that human words could not describe the sights, sounds, and feelings he encountered in heaven. When he was able to read the Bible again and read about heaven, he totally understood what was being described.[1]

In his second book, *Heaven Is Real: Lessons on Earthly Joy*, Don writes the following:

> In the past when I read passages about heaven, I didn't know if they were literal or symbolic. It didn't matter to me on earth. But now that I have been there, I can report, those verses in Revelation refer to literal streets of gold. Every person I saw in my brief trip to heaven was totally healthy. I can tell people about heaven, a joyously perfect eternity, and about God's grace, but until they experience those things for themselves, they have to grasp them by faith. But one day, I remind them, heaven will become a reality.[2]

God has prepared an indescribable life for us in eternity. Yet, until the day that he chooses to take us there, we must live and walk by faith. What greater purpose is there than to invest our lives in helping ensure that others will one day see those streets of gold!

Prayer

Glorious Father, I can hardly imagine what heaven must be like. Perhaps if I thought about it more often, I would not be so consumed with the challenges and difficulties of life here on earth. Please help me live with an eternal perspective, knowing that the best is yet to come. You must want us to think about that since you take the time in your Word to tell us about it. Thank you for loving us so much that you would encourage us with this reality and give us hope eternal. In Jesus's name I pray, amen.

FROM THE DEVOTION ABOVE I HAVE IDENTIFIED . . .

The lie I believe:

The truth I now receive:

☐ ☐ ☐ I practiced healthy self-talk today (one to three times).

My key personal statement is:

☐ ☐ ☐ I have repeated that message at least three times today.

☐ I have written my personal statement above on an index card or in a journal that I can continue to read if I need renewal in this area.

Nourish Your Body—You Gotta Have Heart

No one is surprised when the out-of-shape, overly stressed fifty-something male executive suffers a heart attack. But when a relatively healthy middle-aged woman drops dead from one, everyone is shocked.

Most women worry more about getting breast cancer than having a heart attack, and yet their risk of the latter is higher. In fact, heart disease claims twice as many women's lives as all forms of cancer combined! In the United States, one woman dies from a heart attack or stroke every single minute. The most alarming fact of all is that 60 percent of women who die suddenly from heart disease had no previous symptoms. What we don't realize is that what we can't see and often can't feel can kill us. One day we are walking around feeling great, and the next day—*boom*—we may die from a heart attack. Now if you are a man reading this section, we already know that *you* are at risk. My point is to alert the women (your wives and daughters) that they are also.

Beneath the surface of our skin, so much is going on. Everything we eat, every little lifestyle habit, is producing good or bad results in the cells of our bodies. Sometimes we get warning signs like being overweight or feeling winded climbing just one flight of stairs. Sometimes we don't. I hope I've caught your attention, not to have you stress out with worry but rather to motivate you to action.

The American Heart Association recommends *daily* vigorous activity to benefit both your circulatory and respiratory systems. Vigorous means that you get your heart pumping at 50 to 75 percent of its maximum rate for at least thirty minutes. You can do that with a variety of aerobic activities like walking, biking, swimming, exercise classes—even energetic dancing. There's so much living to do—eat and exercise for health to keep that heart pumping for years to come!

DAILY JOURNAL & LOG

My unhealthy habit(s) is diminishing and my new habits are increasing in the following ways:

Nutrition and Fat Management

I ate for maximum energy and health today in the following ways:

- ☐ By drinking 4 to 6 ounces of water most waking hours.
- ☐ By eating protein and/or fiber at breakfast.
- ☐ By eating 3 to 4 vegetables.
- ☐ By eating 2 to 3 servings of fruits, whole grains, or nuts.

☐ By eating 5 to 6 snacks or small meals.

☐ By eating less from bags and boxes.

☐ By eating only when I was hungry.

☐ By eating 20 to 50 percent less food than usual in the last 4 hours of the day.

☐ By eating no more than 10 percent "empty" calories.

Rest and Regeneration

Last night I slept ____________ hours.

The quality of my sleep was: _________________

Tonight I will ______________________________ to ensure I get quality rest.

Today I managed my stress by:

Tomorrow I will unwind and relax by:

☐ I practiced deep breathing today for relaxation and health.

Fitness

☐ Today I did my minimum 10 minutes of exercise.

I exceeded the minimum by _____________________

Tomorrow I will improve or maintain my fitness by:

Thoughts for Today

day 37

Nourish Your Spirit—The Steadfast Mind

> You will keep in perfect peace him whose mind is steadfast, because he trusts in you.
>
> Isaiah 26:3

Steadfast, unwavering, resolute, persistent, committed, dedicated, firm, unfaltering, dependable, loyal, faithful, reliable, trustworthy, and *constant* are words that describe the mind that God wants you to have in relationship to his faithfulness and truth. When our mind is steadfast, our heart is at peace despite the storm that may be swirling about us. Like the quiet in the eye of a hurricane, a person who keeps her focus intent on the Lord is sheltered in his powerful arms from the anxieties of life.

If you know Christ as your personal Savior, what is the worst thing that can ever happen to you? Think seriously about this question. You may experience loss, pain, and concern for loved ones. But all pain will cease, all heartbreak will vanish, and all tears will be wiped away in heaven. Our life here on earth is like a grain of sand in the ocean of time. We will spend eons more time in heaven (an eternity) than we ever will on earth. One day this life will be a distant memory. In fact, who even knows what we will remember since there is total joy in heaven. Our reality will be complete, yet the pain of the past will have vanished.

In fact, to give you perspective about how we are to think about our troubles in this life, read what Peter said in 1 Peter 5:10 (NASB):

> After you have suffered for a little while, the God of all grace, who called you to His eternal glory in Christ, will Himself perfect, confirm, strengthen and establish you.

That "little while" that Peter mentions is actually this lifetime. Think about all the things that we stress and strain over. We let our unhealthy habits get in the way of dynamic living. We let our unhealthy thoughts distract us from the glorious God who wants to shower us with his love and encourage us with the hope of heaven. When we are steadfast and in perfect peace, we cannot be shaken. Spend some time every day worshipping God for who he is and what he has done. When we set our mind on that which is dependable, faithful, and trustworthy—Jesus Christ—our lives take on a whole new vitality.

Prayer

Father, please forgive me for taking my eyes off you too often and seeing life inaccurately. Help me to have a steadfast mind that interprets every single thing through a heart that trusts you completely. As I work toward a healthier mind and body, please remind me that a healthy spirit will ensure that I am all that and more. In Jesus's powerful name I pray, amen.

FROM THE DEVOTION ABOVE I HAVE IDENTIFIED . . .

The lie I believe:

The truth I now receive:

☐ ☐ ☐ I practiced healthy self-talk today (one to three times).

My key personal statement is:

☐ ☐ ☐ I have repeated that message at least three times today.

☐ I have written my personal statement above on an index card or in a journal that I can continue to read if I need renewal in this area.

Nourish Your Body—Ultraclean Living Backfires

Experts are reporting that many allergies and immune-system diseases have doubled, tripled, or even quadrupled in the last thirty to forty years. Some studies confirm that more than half of the U.S. population has at least one allergy. Many researchers suspect the increase may be due to changes in modern living to include the "hygiene hypothesis," which blames growing up in increasingly sterile homes as the problem. Others have pointed to changes in diet, air pollution, and even the rise in obesity and sedentary lifestyles.

Interestingly, the rise in allergies and immune-system diseases are only showing up in highly developed countries in Europe and North America. The illnesses have steadily increased in other countries as they have become more advanced.

This is what health expert Dr. Joseph Mercola says about this issue:

> As society in general becomes more "sterile," it is causing real problems for your immune system, which is becoming increasingly unable to differentiate between real threats and harmless things like pollen and dust-bunnies.
>
> Think about it: how many people do you know who carry a bottle of antibacterial hand sanitizer with them wherever they go? Meanwhile, you're exposed to antibiotics, in your food and by prescription, while most of the food supply is pasteurized or otherwise treated to remove both good and bad bacteria.

> And this is the key: while everyone was so busy killing all of those "germs," they didn't stop to think about what this would mean for the future generations. Children are now growing up without being exposed to the bacteria, viruses, and parasites that have existed throughout the world—even in developed countries like the United States—since the beginning of time.
>
> To some extent, this is a good thing. But to children's immune systems, which are not being exposed to bacteria and viruses like they were in the past, it results in an excessive immune response against a routine thing, like a peanut, resulting in allergies and autoimmune diseases.[1]

While "clean living" is certainly a good thing, we must be wise and not take this to an extreme. We also need to stop pressuring our doctors to write prescriptions for antibiotics every time we have a sniffle or a cough. They should not be giving in to these requests, but unfortunately sometimes they do, which results in increasingly resistant strains of bacteria and a much bigger problem for all of us. Don't feel you have to avoid every germ on the planet. Let your kids play in the dirt. Yes, we do need to wash our hands after using the restroom and when in contact with sick people. But that old "ten second" rule for food dropped on the floor not being contaminated is a good one to keep. Our bodies get strengthened by small doses of bacteria. Let's not be afraid to live in the "real" world and leave our hand sanitizer behind on occasion.

DAILY JOURNAL & LOG

My unhealthy habit(s) is diminishing and my new habits are increasing in the following ways:

Nutrition and Fat Management

I ate for maximum energy and health today in the following ways:

- ☐ By drinking 4 to 6 ounces of water most waking hours.
- ☐ By eating protein and/or fiber at breakfast.
- ☐ By eating 3 to 4 vegetables.
- ☐ By eating 2 to 3 servings of fruits, whole grains, or nuts.
- ☐ By eating 5 to 6 snacks or small meals.
- ☐ By eating less from bags and boxes.
- ☐ By eating only when I was hungry.
- ☐ By eating 20 to 50 percent less food than usual in the last 4 hours of the day.
- ☐ By eating no more than 10 percent "empty" calories.

Rest and Regeneration

Last night I slept ____________ hours.

The quality of my sleep was: ________________

Tonight I will ______________________________ to ensure I get quality rest.

Today I managed my stress by:

Tomorrow I will unwind and relax by:

☐ I practiced deep breathing today for relaxation and health.

Fitness

☐ Today I did my minimum 10 minutes of exercise.

I exceeded the minimum by ____________________

Tomorrow I will improve or maintain my fitness by:

Thoughts for Today

day 38

Nourish Your Spirit—Faith of a Child

> And without faith it is impossible to please God, because anyone who comes to him must believe that he exists and that he rewards those who earnestly seek him.
>
> Hebrews 11:6

One Sunday morning many years ago, when my son, Jesse, was only four, we overslept and were going to be late for church. I called out to wake him as I entered his room, "Jesse, it's time to get up, it's Sunday. We're going to church. Jesus is waiting!"

Jesus is waiting. It just slipped out innocently. I had no idea the impact it would have on our entire day!

The first words out of his froggy little throat were, "He *is*? Jesus is at church today?"

"Of course, sweetheart, Jesus is always at church," I responded.

"He *is*?" he replied in wonder.

"Well, yes, Jesse. Jesus is everywhere. And he especially likes to be at church. So, let's get going or we'll be late!" I answered in some exasperation as I prodded him out of bed. Ten minutes later he appeared in my bathroom with sunglasses on, and I asked him why he was wearing them. "So I can see Jesus better when we get to church," he replied.

"Honey, you can't see Jesus with your eyes . . . he's in your heart."

"But, I want to *see* Jesus!" Jesse cried out.

Oh, the challenges of explaining the spiritual dimension to little ones! All morning at church, Jesse was peeking around corners and "sleuthing" into rooms like an espionage agent trying to sneak up on Jesus. I think that he had the impression that Jesus was playing some spiritual version of hide-and-seek. He just couldn't understand why Jesus would not reveal himself physically.

Our usual routine after church is a quick trip to Starbucks. As my husband and I loaded him into the backseat, he continued his quest. "Will Jesus be at Starbucks too, Dad?" he asked.

"Well, I guess he will be if we're there, because he never leaves us!" my husband answered.

After coffee, we took a quick jaunt into the local drugstore before heading home. "Is Jesus here too?" Jesse asked again. We continued to try our best to explain that Jesus is always with us because we have asked him into our hearts and received forgiveness for our sins through his death on the cross. Jesse said, "I know Jesus is in my heart. But can I pull him out from under my bones?"

In a cynical world, it is so refreshing to watch the innocent discovery of a child seeking spiritual truth. As adults, we become desensitized to the miracles of God. The technology of television, movies, and computers has dulled our senses to the real miracles of life. And now the true spiritual dimension and miracles of the Bible are put in the same mental file cabinets often subconsciously labeled "fiction." Our minds have difficulty conceiving the intangible unless we get some spiritual help.

The Bible says that we will find God when we seek him with all of our hearts. He is real. He *is* tangible. No, not with our physical senses, but his Spirit will connect with ours when we seek him with faith like a child. Jesus said that anyone who will not receive the kingdom of God like a little child will never enter it (Luke 18:17).

And so, I marveled at the faith of my curious, knee-scraped little guy who never gave up all Sunday looking for Jesus. We pulled into the garage, gathered up our packages, and helped Jesse out of the car when we finally got home that afternoon. He was the first of us to reach the back door into the house. Pulling it open, he yelled at the top of his little lungs, "Jesus, we're home!"

Jesus was there waiting for us . . . as he always is. So Jesse and I just plopped down on the steps leading upstairs and had a little talk with him. We told him how much we loved him for dying for our sins. We thanked him for loving us that much. We told him we could feel his presence even if we couldn't see him. I took a little peek at Jesse during our prayer time. He had one eye open watching for Jesus.

Whenever you feel far from God, just call out to him like Jesse did. And he will respond . . . when you have the faith of a child.

Prayer

Heavenly Father, oh how I want to have faith like a child. Sometimes my actions reveal that my faith is weak. I pray that you will forgive me for that and help me to seek you with a heart of expectation, knowing that you are always with me and that you love me with an everlasting love. Lord, I know my greatest reward is the sense of power and peace I have to face all of life's challenges when my faith in you is strong. Help me to grow in faith and glorify you. Amen.

FROM THE DEVOTION ABOVE I HAVE IDENTIFIED . . .

The lie I believe:

The truth I now receive:

☐ ☐ ☐ I practiced healthy self-talk today (one to three times).

My key personal statement is:

☐ ☐ ☐ I have repeated that message at least three times today.

☐ I have written my personal statement above on an index card or in a journal that I can continue to read if I need renewal in this area.

Nourish Your Body—Fat-Fighting Ideas

Put on your bathing suit every day in front of a full length mirror and ask yourself this question: "Do I really want to store extra fat on my body?"

Drink a large glass of water (always a good thing) before going to a special dinner or buffet. It not only fills you up but also reminds you of your goal to eat with purpose.

Get a reality check: most cookies, candies, and other treats are at least 150 calories per ounce. That's more than a full tablespoon of butter. Keep that in mind and tell yourself, *I can be fully satisfied with just one or two morsels.*

Stabilize your blood sugar to decrease cravings. A lean, healthy breakfast and lunch that each have at least 15 grams of protein and 5–10 grams of fiber (and no empty calories) will give you great energy and balance to withstand temptations more effectively.

Stock up on healthy snacks that will help you say no to the goodies and treats that really aren't your favorites anyway. Healthy energy bars will give you a sweet fix and still keep you on track. Fruit, veggies, and nuts (in moderation) are always great options.

Practice the ten-minute delay rule. Every time you have an urge to try one more cookie or your favorite fun food, just make yourself wait ten minutes. Then, if you really still want it, go ahead and take one small portion. Then wait another ten minutes for the next bite. If nothing else, you will eat considerably fewer calories.

Always offer to bring a healthy option to any dinner or party you attend. This will allow you to eat a bit more volume of something you know will fill you up without all the fat and calories.

DAILY JOURNAL & LOG

My unhealthy habit(s) is diminishing and my new habits are increasing in the following ways:

Nutrition and Fat Management

I ate for maximum energy and health today in the following ways:

- ☐ By drinking 4 to 6 ounces of water most waking hours.
- ☐ By eating protein and/or fiber at breakfast.
- ☐ By eating 3 to 4 vegetables.
- ☐ By eating 2 to 3 servings of fruits, whole grains, or nuts.
- ☐ By eating 5 to 6 snacks or small meals.
- ☐ By eating less from bags and boxes.
- ☐ By eating only when I was hungry.

- ☐ By eating 20 to 50 percent less food than usual in the last 4 hours of the day.
- ☐ By eating no more than 10 percent "empty" calories.

Rest and Regeneration

Last night I slept ____________ hours.

The quality of my sleep was: __________________

Tonight I will ________________________________ to ensure I get quality rest.

Today I managed my stress by:

Tomorrow I will unwind and relax by:

☐ I practiced deep breathing today for relaxation and health.

Fitness

☐ Today I did my minimum 10 minutes of exercise.

I exceeded the minimum by ______________________

Tomorrow I will improve or maintain my fitness by:

Thoughts for Today

day 39

Nourish Your Spirit—Obsessed with God

> His divine power has given us everything we need for life and godliness through our knowledge of him who called us by his own glory and goodness.
>
> 2 Peter 1:3

If you heard someone say, "She is such a godly woman," what would come to your mind? *Godliness* is a word that can be easily misinterpreted. It may conjure up images of a very religious person who is extremely self-controlled in their actions. Or perhaps we think of a person like Mother Teresa, who totally sacrificed her life for the poor, and say to ourselves, "I could never live a godly life like she did."

Many of us have the misconception that godliness is realized by keeping a set of rules and that God is pleased with our self-control. We believe if we give up things for God, we will receive more blessings. This attitude has us living in fear of failing God and displeasing others and thus motivates us to toe the line. While Mother Teresa truly was a godly woman, her godliness came out of her love for God and others, rather than a religious obligation.

Because we have freedom in Christ, the motivation restraining our behavior should be love, not fear. We may choose certain behaviors or restrictions so as to protect our souls or that of our Christian brothers and sisters. When we are overflowing with love, we will also choose the best and joyfully sacrifice our own rights when we understand the liberty we have in Christ. True spirituality is the surrender of our heart to the Lord. It frees us from the bondage of potential failure.

The verse above says that God in his divine power has already given us everything we need to live a godly life. It says that our knowledge of Christ is our motivation. When we look upon his glory and goodness, we should be moved beyond words and so grateful that our greatest desire in life is to bring him glory. I love how my pastor defines godliness. He says that it is being obsessed with God and the things of God.

I've been obsessed with food in my life. I've also been obsessed with exercise, love, and sometimes even accomplishment. I don't know about you, but I really want to be totally obsessed with God alone. If God has given us all we need to be godly, then we must do our part to grow in the knowledge of Christ. If we turn our attention intently on him, he will transform us day by day.

Prayer

Father God, when I look at the glory and goodness of Christ, how can I help but be transformed? Yet some days I find myself more obsessed with my plans and concerns than with you. I desire to become a godly person. Please help me to have pure motives and to become obsessed with loving you fully. In Jesus's name, amen.

FROM THE DEVOTION ABOVE I HAVE IDENTIFIED . . .

The lie I believe:

The truth I now receive:

☐ ☐ ☐ I practiced healthy self-talk today (one to three times).

My key personal statement is:

☐ ☐ ☐ I have repeated that message at least three times today.

☐ I have written my personal statement above on an index card or in a journal that I can continue to read if I need renewal in this area.

Nourish Your Body—Too Much or Too Little of a Good Thing

We've all heard and believed the old cliché "If you don't use it, you'll lose it." Of course it means if we don't use our body fully, it will degenerate. Our muscles and bones atrophy if they aren't being stimulated regularly. Our cardiovascular and respiratory systems become sluggish and potentially diseased and we lose energy and vitality when we don't move our bodies in healthful ways.

But, the opposite is true as well. If we overuse our bodies with too much of the same activity day after day, it can result in injuries and chronic pain. This can happen to runners and elite athletes. It can also happen to sedentary folks. Using even the smallest body part too much can cause injury. In this age of sedentary living and desk jobs, you see more and more people with neck strain, carpal tunnel, and lower back issues from sitting too much at their computers. Even talking on the phone too much can create tension and inflammation of the upper back and shoulders. The list goes on and on.

The solution is to modify all activity so each body part gets both stimulated and rested sufficiently. Stretching is also an important factor in keeping the body in balance. We need to counteract that which we do most often and in turn move and condition the body parts that rarely get used.

If you drive or sit at a desk much of your day, it is essential to get up and move around at least once an hour. Roll your shoulders back and stretch your quadricep muscles by pulling your heel toward your buttocks with one hand and holding that position for at least thirty seconds on each side. Take a short walk to the other side of your home or office. Simply move in opposite ways of your most common activities.

In sports, it is important to mix up your workouts to avoid injuries and also maximize the benefits of your favorite activities. If you do the same thing every day, over time you will burn 25 percent less calories and get less fitness gain overall. For example, if you love running, add in swimming, weight training, or biking at least twice a week.

Our body tells us when we've been doing too much of something and asks us in the form of aches and pains to treat it differently. When we listen and give it what it needs, it will usually bounce back readily. Stay active, yet be smart. Too much of a good thing is simply too much. And too little of a good thing will age you prematurely. It's all about balance!

DAILY JOURNAL & LOG

My unhealthy habit(s) is diminishing and my new habits are increasing in the following ways:

Nutrition and Fat Management

I ate for maximum energy and health today in the following ways:

- ☐ By drinking 4 to 6 ounces of water most waking hours.
- ☐ By eating protein and/or fiber at breakfast.
- ☐ By eating 3 to 4 vegetables.
- ☐ By eating 2 to 3 servings of fruits, whole grains, or nuts.

☐ By eating 5 to 6 snacks or small meals.

☐ By eating less from bags and boxes.

☐ By eating only when I was hungry.

☐ By eating 20 to 50 percent less food than usual in the last 4 hours of the day.

☐ By eating no more than 10 percent "empty" calories.

Rest and Regeneration

Last night I slept ____________ hours.

The quality of my sleep was: ________________

Tonight I will ______________________________ to ensure I get quality rest.

Today I managed my stress by:

Tomorrow I will unwind and relax by:

☐ I practiced deep breathing today for relaxation and health.

Fitness

☐ Today I did my minimum 10 minutes of exercise.

I exceeded the minimum by _____________________

Tomorrow I will improve or maintain my fitness by:

Thoughts for Today

day 40

Nourish Your Spirit—The One Thing

> "Love the Lord your God with all your heart and with all your soul and with all your mind." This is the first and greatest commandment. And the second is like it: "Love your neighbor as yourself." All the Law and the Prophets hang on these two commandments.
>
> Matthew 22:37–40

Years ago in my days as a corporate marketing manager, I facilitated a business course for the "Fortune 100" company that employed me. The program was from what would become a hugely bestselling book called *The Seven Habits of Highly Effective People* by Stephen Covey. It taught time-honored principles that helped people become their best in both their private and business lives. The teaching was sound and effective. My years in that world were both stressful and exhausting as the expectation to excel always trumped home and family. I realized the price I was paying for a great income was too high. After eight years, I gave up the financial benefits and never looked back. God rewarded me in much greater ways that money cannot buy. Yet, years later after I had become a Christian author and speaker, one key question from Covey's teaching kept popping into my mind for some reason. It was from his chapter "Putting First Things First," and it said:

> What one thing could you do (that you aren't doing right now) on a regular basis that would make a tremendous positive difference in your life?[1]

As a recovering type A, I thought this question had a lot of potential to help people get focused. However, I also knew that as Christians, we need to submit all of our plans and goals to God. It seemed to me that if I could change that question a bit, I could help myself and others move closer to God's purpose for all the dimensions of our lives. So, I rewrote the question to look like this:

> Based on God's Word, what one thing could you focus on daily that would make a tremendous and God-honoring difference in your life?

Soon I was speaking all over the country on my new topic that I called "The One Thing," asking people to ask themselves this question in not only their entire life but in each specific dimension to include their physical, material, relational, mental, and vocational areas. Using scriptural principals as a guide, I showed women how to identify their areas of weakness and even sin and refocus their attention to the "one thing" that would make the biggest difference in that area. My last life area to cover was always the physical dimension, and my key Scripture for that area is our Scripture for today. In essence, it is the only Scripture we really need when it comes to finding true focus in life.

The religious leaders of Jesus's time wanted to trip him up and prove that he was an ineffective teacher and not the Son of God whom he declared himself to be. So, when the Pharisees asked him what was the greatest commandment of all, Jesus answered that it was to "love the Lord your God with all your heart and with all your soul and with all your mind." But he didn't stop; he went on to say, "And the second is like it: Love your neighbor as yourself." And then he made the most profound comment, saying, "All the Law and the Prophets hang on these two commandments." In essence if we love God with our entire being—if that is our primary life purpose—and if we secondly love others as we love ourselves, every single commandment of God will be fulfilled. This is the most profound thing. It is the "one thing" that deserves all of our heart, mind, and soul.

If you want to overcome bad habits, if you want a transformed life, if you want great peace and joy, you need to pay attention to this "one thing." God is a jealous God. Like a husband who sees his wife being distracted by the attention of another man, God too is jealous of everything that takes our eyes off him. He gave absolutely everything to redeem our souls and bring us back into beautiful intimacy with him for all eternity. And all he asks is for us to love him completely and love each other. When that above all is our "one thing," all else will be fulfilled.

Prayer

Almighty God, you alone are worthy of praise. You alone are worthy of my first thoughts, my first love, and my first energy. I am so weak without you. Please forgive me when I don't give you my best. You are the "one thing" worthy of my attention and love. Help me to become the person you want me to be, whole in your love, so full that your love overflows from me to the others in my life. In Jesus's name I pray, amen.

FROM THE DEVOTION ABOVE I HAVE IDENTIFIED . . .

The lie I believe:

The truth I now receive:

☐ ☐ ☐ I practiced healthy self-talk today (one to three times).

My key personal statement is:

☐ ☐ ☐ I have repeated that message at least three times today.

- ☐ I have written my personal statement above on an index card or in a journal that I can continue to read if I need renewal in this area.

Nourish Your Body—God's Perfect Foods

I've often looked at a banana, kiwi, or almost any of God's beautiful fruits and wondered how someone could not believe in an intimate personal Creator. His packaging is perfect, each fruit dense with life-giving nutrients. Amazing! Man will never be able to replicate what God has done perfectly.

Plant foods provide us with fabulous phytochemicals that dramatically impact our health in multitudes of ways. For example, garlic contains a substance called allicin, a natural antibiotic. Indoles can be found in cabbage and broccoli. These help protect against cancer. Dried beans and peas are full of saponins, which help lower cholesterol and protect against osteoporosis. Tomatoes contain the richest source of the phytochemical lycopene, the pigment that gives them their red color. One glass of tomato juice has the lycopene of forty tomato slices!

Every second of your life, your cells are bombarded by dangerous particles called free radicals. Free radicals are molecules that are missing an electron, which they attempt to snatch from any other molecule available. In a split second, they can alter your DNA in ways that cause cancer, change LDL cholesterol (the bad cholesterol) so it sticks to artery walls, or damage collagen and make skin wrinkle prone. The oxidation effect can be compared to the browning of a cut apple or the rust on a car. You cannot see or feel the damage of these free radicals until many cells are compromised and disease or premature aging results.

Fortunately, you can fight back. Load your diet with antioxidants—the natural zappers of free radicals—by eating lots of fruits and vegetables. The bright and dark color of fruits and vegetables generally means they are richer in nutrients. For example, buy red grapes instead of green, red cabbage instead of green, and romaine lettuce instead of iceberg.

Here's an interesting fact about antioxidants. Tufts University in Boston and scientist Ronald Prior, PhD, recommend adding a half cup of blueberries to your diet every day (a dramatic increase over our current average intake of about two and a half cups a year). With a half cup of blueberries, you can practically double the amount of antioxidants most Americans get in one day. Blueberries beat out thirty-nine other common fruits and vegetables in antioxidant power—even kale, strawberries, spinach, and broccoli! Wow!

Buy produce at different stages of ripeness so there will always be some ready for you to eat. Splurge on prepackaged salads, fruits, and vegetables. They might be a little more expensive, but they're time efficient and you're more likely to eat the produce before it goes bad in your refrigerator. Just think of it as an investment in your health. Make it a practice to buy one new kind of healthful food every time you go to the market.

DAILY JOURNAL & LOG

My unhealthy habit(s) is diminishing and my new habits are increasing in the following ways:

Nutrition and Fat Management

I ate for maximum energy and health today in the following ways:

☐ By drinking 4 to 6 ounces of water most waking hours.

☐ By eating protein and/or fiber at breakfast.

☐ By eating 3 to 4 vegetables.

☐ By eating 2 to 3 servings of fruits, whole grains, or nuts.

☐ By eating 5 to 6 snacks or small meals.

☐ By eating less from bags and boxes.

☐ By eating only when I was hungry.

☐ By eating 20 to 50 percent less food than usual in the last 4 hours of the day.

☐ By eating no more than 10 percent "empty" calories.

Rest and Regeneration

Last night I slept ____________ hours.

The quality of my sleep was: __________________

Tonight I will _______________________________ to ensure I get quality rest.

Today I managed my stress by:

Tomorrow I will unwind and relax by:

☐ I practiced deep breathing today for relaxation and health.

Fitness

☐ Today I did my minimum 10 minutes of exercise.

I exceeded the minimum by ______________________

Tomorrow I will improve or maintain my fitness by:

Thoughts for Today

the journey continues

The day I graduated from nursing school, I felt such a great sense of satisfaction and accomplishment. And then a few months later when I passed the grueling state board exams, I was ready to go out into the world as a professional registered nurse. And yet, the truth be told, my real education had only just begun. Each day I would learn new skills and acquire greater knowledge. Eventually as a veteran labor and delivery nurse, I would teach what I knew to nurses with less experience.

Your forty-day journey has been an important one, and if you've come this far, you have laid an important foundation for lasting change. Yet, your daily work has just begun. The purposeful use of self-talk, daily introspection, and logging are all very good tools to continue as you lock in permanently the changes you have begun. And of course, meditating on God's truth is something that will grow and sustain us daily for a lifetime.

Many years ago I was introduced to Oswald Chambers's powerful devotional *My Utmost for His Highest*, from which I quoted in several places in this book. The first year I read it, it was so life-changing that I read it every day for almost seven years. Each year, I seemed to get something more from the same devotion I had read many times before. I encourage you to go back to the chapters and daily readings in this book that spoke most powerfully to you and review them again and again. As I have already explained, it is the repetition of good thoughts that burns a permanent groove into our minds.

Continue the good, healthy habits you started by using whatever tools I have taught you that help you in maintaining a consistent healthy walk. I have also listed below a few of the tools I use with my clients, some that I have already mentioned, that are available to you on my website. If you use the code "CHCL" if you choose to order anything, it will automatically give you a 10 percent discount on all my resources until January 2010 to include nutritional supplements, books, and CDs that I have not listed below. You can visit my website at www.dannademetre.com.

I wish you many blessings on your journey,

Danna

a few recommended resources

Change Your Habits, Change Your Life Healthy Self-Talk CD
Caltrac Activity Monitor

Scale Down Products:
Scale Down book
Scale Down workbook
Scale Down—Live It Up audio series (6 sessions)
Scale Down—Live It Up DVD series (6 sessions)
Healthy Self-Talk CD
Leader's Guide
Remember to use code CHCL when ordering!

the perfect love

Countless love stories have ended with heartbreaking conclusions. A man and a woman who were destined to be together find each other, fall passionately in love, and then some tragic situation tears them apart, leaving each with a gaping hole in their heart for the rest of their lives. Each and every human who has ever walked this planet has the potential to find perfect love—a love that will never be tragically pulled from you, a love that will never betray you, a love that will never die and leave you alone. That perfect love is Jesus Christ. If before reading this book, you did not know Christ, it is my prayer that you have come to see a glimpse of him in these pages and begun to understand that he loves you personally and intimately.

Even other religions call Jesus a prophet and a good teacher. Yet he is so much more. He claimed to be the Son of God. If this is not true, how could someone call a person who made insane claims a good teacher or even a prophet? Jesus is either who he says he is or he is a liar.

Many people have sought to disprove the deity of Christ. Men like Lee Strobel, an investigative reporter and staunch atheist, went about his quest with all the skills he had used professionally, only to come to a shocking conclusion: Jesus is who he said he was—God in the flesh. When he read the accounts and searched the historical records, there was not doubt that Jesus Christ walked the earth. And the reports from eyewitnesses were all consistent. Jesus died and was buried for three days . . . and then he rose again to newness of life. Lee writes of his powerful and life-changing journey in his book *A Case for Christ.*[1]

My point in writing these last few words is not to convince you by words that Jesus Christ is the only way to heaven—the only way to intimacy with God. My point is to say this: if Jesus Christ is not yet your Savior, if you do not *know* that you *know* that you *know* him, then please pray for him to reveal himself to you fully. You may doubt if what I have said is true. Test it for yourself. Everyone must make a decision about Jesus. Making no decision at all is actually rejection. If there is even a chance he is who he says he is, doesn't it make sense to find this out now rather than after your death?

Moving from hearing to knowing, and knowing to believing can be the longest journey ever known. But it is God who draws a seeking heart to himself and reveals his truth in supernatural ways. If you humbly submit yourself to God and seek him with all of your heart . . . you will find him. He says so in his Word. He will turn the "facts" you have heard about Jesus into transforming truth that penetrates your heart and transforms your life.

As I write these words, it is Easter weekend, the time we commemorate the greatest single act of love ever performed in the history of humanity. That love gift was given for every person who has ever been born. Jesus Christ came to the earth in the body of a man for the sole purpose of dying for our sins . . . for your sins. If you were the only person alive, he would have done that just for you. If you believe that fact and accept his free gift of forgiveness, you will be saved and have eternal life. It's that simple.

> For God so loved the world that he gave his only Son, that whoever believes in him shall not perish but have eternal life.
>
> John 3:16

Don't let your love story have a tragic ending. The most perfect love in the universe is reaching out to embrace you, heal you, love you. Won't you open your heart and let him in?

notes

Chapter 2: Change Your Mind

1. Bob George, *Classic Christianity* (Eugene, OR: Harvest House, 1989), 9.
2. Max Lucado, *A Heart Like Jesus*, taken from www.smileofachild.org.
3. Oswald Chambers, *My Utmost for His Highest* (Grand Rapids: Discovery House, 1963), 131.
4. Ibid., 328.
5. William Backus, *The Healing Power of the Christian Mind* (Minneapolis: Bethany, 1996), 133.
6. Ibid., 14, 72.

Chapter 3: The Battle of the Flesh

1. David Needham, *Birthright* (Sisters, OR: Multnomah, 1979), 98.
2. George, *Classic Christianity*, 137–38.
3. Elyse Fitzpatrick, *Idols of the Heart* (Wheaton: Tyndale, 2001), 15.

Chapter 4: Change Your Habits

1. James F. Balch, MD, *The Super Anti-Oxidants* (New York: M. Evans and Company, 1998), 6.
2. Francisco Contreras, MD, *The Hope of Living Long and Well* (Lake Mary, FL: Siloam Press/Strang Communications, 2000), 93.
3. Dr. Joseph Mercola, taken from his website, Mercola.com; used by permission.
4. Sylvia Lange, recording artist and speaker, can be contacted at www.sylvialange.com.
5. Reprinted from *The Twelve Steps for Christians: A Spiritual Journey, a Working Guide for Healing* (Curtis, WA: RPI Publishing, 1988), 31, 43, 55, 69, 97, 109, 123, 139, 153, 167, 197, 211.

Chapter 5: A Forty-Day Strategy Toward Permanent Change

1. Chambers, *My Utmost for His Highest*, 210.

Day 6: Nourish Your Body—Rusting and Rotting

1. Balch, *The Super Anti-Oxidants*, 6.

Day 7: Nourish Your Body—Fitness Tips

1. Heather Dillinger, an IDEA personal trainer, Health.com, January/February 2008.

Day 10: Nourish Your Spirit—Body on Loan from God

1. Chambers, *My Utmost for His Highest*, 131.

Day 11: Nourish Your Spirit—The Beginning of Wisdom

1. Michael Burlingame, ed., *Lincoln Observed: The Civil War Dispatches of Noah Brooks* (Baltimore: Johns Hopkins University Press, 1988), 210.
2. www.encouragementonline.net.

Day 12: Nourish Your Body—More Fat Facts

1. Jordan Rubin, *The Maker's Diet* (Lake Mary, FL: Siloam Press, 2004), 135.

Day 14: Nourish Your Body—Health Tidbits You Can Use

1. Jordan Rubin, *The Great Physician's Rx for Health and Wellness* (Nashville: Thomas Nelson, 2005), 41.

Day 17: Nourish Your Spirit—Seize the Day

1. www.motherteresauniv.org.

Day 17: Nourish Your Body—Acid-Alkaline Balance

1. Dr. Christopher Vassey, *Acid-Alkaline Diet for Optimum Health* (Rochester, VT, 1999), 4.

Day 18: Nourish Your Body—Nix the Artificial

1. Mercola, Mercola.com; used by permission.

Day 21: Nourish Your Spirit—Choosing the Best from All the Good

1. Edwin Louis Cole, *Profiles in Courageous Manhood* (Tulsa: Albury, 1998), 25.

Day 22: Nourish Your Spirit—Joyful . . . Prayerful . . . Thankful

1. www.sermonillustrations.com.

Day 23: Nourish Your Body—Fasting for Health

1. Rubin, *The Great Physician's Rx for Health and Wellness*, 41–42.

Day 24: Nourish Your Body—Stress Kills

1. Marcia Ramsland, *Simplify Your Time: Stop Running and Start Living* (Nashville: Thomas Nelson, 2006), xi.

Day 28: Nourish Your Body—Thyroid News You Can Use

1. Amanda Edleman, registered pharmacist, Life Wellness Pharmacy, Carlsbad, CA.

Day 32: Nourish Your Body—Healthy Gums . . . Healthy Heart

1. www.perio.org/consumer/bacteria.htm.

Day 33: Nourish Your Body—Exercise Your Mind

1. www.sfn.org/index.ctm?pagename=news_11082003d.

Day 36: Nourish Your Spirit—No Eye Has Seen

1. Don Piper with Cecil Murphey, *90 Minutes in Heaven* (Grand Rapids: Revell, 2004).
2. Don Piper, *Heaven Is Real* (London: Berkley Publishing Group, 2007), 24–25.

Day 37: Nourish Your Body—Ultraclean Living Backfires

1. Mercola, Mercola.com; used by permission.

Day 40: Nourish Your Spirit—The One Thing

1. Stephen Covey, *The Seven Habits of Highly Effective People* (New York: Fireside, 1989).

The Perfect Love

1. Lee Strobel, *The Case for Christ* (Grand Rapids: Zondervan, 1998).

Self-described as a "work in progress," **Danna Demetre** has learned how to find deep satisfaction by putting first things first in each area of her life. A survivor of marital infidelity, the heartbreak of rebellious children, the paralysis of unrelenting panic attacks and prolonged bondage to food, she has personally discovered that God's Word is truly "living and active and more powerful than a two-edged sword." In fact, that sword is much like a precision surgical knife that when turned on ourselves cuts out the lies we believe and replaces them with truth.

In addition to over twenty-five years in the health and fitness industries, Danna was a former radio talk show host and continues to be a sought-after media guest. She is a popular international speaker and author of several books, including *Scale Down* with its companion church curriculum. Danna lives in San Diego with her husband, Lew, and their adopted grandson, Jesse. For more information visit: www.dannademetre.com.